LIFE AFTER 60:
THE GOLDEN YEARS

THE FACING PROJECT PRESS

An imprint of The Facing Project

Muncie, Indiana 47305

facingproject.com

First published in the United States of America by The Facing Project Press, an imprint of The Facing Project and division of The Facing Project Gives Inc., 2022.

Copyright © 2022. All Rights Reserved.

No part of this book may be reproduced, stored in a retrieval system, transmitted in any form by any means (electronic, mechanical, photocopying, recording, scanning, or otherwise) or used in any manner without written permission of the Publisher (except for the use of quotations in a book review). Requests to the Publisher for permission should be sent via email to: howdy@facingproject.com. Please include "Permission" in the subject line.

First paperback edition November 2022

Cover design by Shantanu Suman

Library of Congress Control Number: 2022939949

ISBN: 978-1-7345581-4-2 (paperback)

ISBN: 978-1-7345581-5-9 (eBook)

Printed in the United States of America

10 9 8 7 6 5 4 3 2 1

Foreword

This Facing Project volume was a lot like life. It was sailing along: storytellers, writers, interviews, composition, and bam! With the onset of COVID 19, everything hit the wall. Before we could move forward with any connection and speed, two years had gone by. Isn't that the way life can be when we least expect it?

But there were stories to be told, lessons to be learned, reflections to be made and an opportunity to look at life after 60 and the golden years. For some seniors they have not been particularly golden. Beset with health problems, loss, and a peculiar sense of unfamiliarity after retirement, the paths for some through the golden years have sometimes been rocky. For others caring for family, loving grandchildren, celebrating friendships, enjoying hobbies, and the busy blur of service and volunteerism have taken them on a whirlwind race while days planned for relaxing and pondering have been filled to the brim.

This Facing Project has allowed us to look at life and war, careers and accomplishments, dementia and illness, strength and bravery, struggle and tenacity, love and respect, all through the eyes of Munsonians ranging in age from 60 to 95. A thread runs through all the stories though: connections, associations, and relationships. It's the same thread showing up as golden strands in all our lives' tapestries.

In 2012 Kelsey Timmerman and J.R. Jamison were volunteers for TEAMwork for Quality Living where I worked. They helped put together stories from people living in poverty to create the first Facing Project, and this important relationship-based storytelling initiative was born. And now, under their leadership, literally hundreds of projects across the US have been launched and, in this case, even paused. But when all is said and done, we all develop links as we face people, their stories and ensuing bravery through life's ventures—sought or unwelcome. And it is in that process that we encounter similarities that bind us together in our humanness.

Molly Ford Flodder
Steering Committee Chair
Life After 60: The Golden Years

Contents

Chapter 1: Connections Along my Pathway — 1

Chapter 2: A Timeless Classic — 5

Chapter 3: Where I'm Supposed to Be — 10

Chapter 4: I'm Busy Retiring—Please Leave a Message! — 13

Chapter 5: The Unforgettable Now — 17

Chapter 6: Freeing the Survivor — 22

Chapter 7: A Life Coach Full of Surprise — 26

Chapter 8: Facing Racism with Help — 30

Chapter 9: The 11th Most Wanted Man in America — 34

Chapter 10: Facing Aging — 38

Chapter 11: I Choose to be Happy; I Choose to be Busy — 42

Chapter 12: Content at 73: Diligent Worker and Vietnam Vet Battles PTSD to Find Joy — 44

Chapter 13: After Kazakhstan — 52

Chapter 14: Honesty Helped When It was My Turn — 57

Chapter 15: Train Ride — 64

Chapter 16: I Was Mad, Real Mad — 68

Chapter 17: Michael Brockley Looks Back on His Life through His Own Words	73
Chapter 18: Fighting Racism with Love	76
Chapter 19: Discovering The Person I've Always Been	80
Chapter 20: Facing the Fight: Systemic Racism in Muncie	86
Chapter 21: Times to Make a Difference	90
Chapter 22: When the Unrest Came to Middletown	96
Chapter 23: A Time for Everything	100
Chapter 24: Learning From Our Children	104
Submitted Bios for Storytellers & Writers	108
Sponsors	112
About The Facing Project	113

Chapter 1: Connections Along My Pathway

Jonathan Mitchell's Story as Told to Molly Flodder

I missed out on an important relationship, and I allowed that absence to shape my early life. Although most of my friends, as I was growing up in western Pennsylvania, had father figures in their lives, I didn't. My mom was a good mom. She worked hard and obtained an RN degree, but it was still a hard life for her, my older sister and me. For my mother to go back to school, we spent several years living in the projects, and as the years passed, I constantly felt different because I was born out of wedlock and because there was no dad in the picture—a real stigma in the mid-60s. Somehow, I felt rejected, sort of like I was being told "God doesn't love you." There was no man to force me to buckle down in school either, so I just sort of drifted along.

That shaped a lot of my growing up years and early adulthood. And, in spite of everything, I was experiencing and allowing myself to go through, I had a sense of calling, a feeling that God had a plan for my life. I started my adult life going to college briefly. Then I joined the Air Force...not exactly a good fit for me. I knocked around for a while, and ended up in Long Island, New York. And because of bad decision-making, I actually ended up homeless for a short time, during which I almost froze to death one night. I went from job to job, and even drove a tractor trailer for a while until a serious injury from a truck accident meant that I was on disability for several years. It even led to a substance abuse problem at one point. At this time, I was determined that life was anything but fair. But I remembered what the "old folk" used to say: "Life isn't fair for anyone."

I continued to feel the pain of rejection during all these years. Which gave me the terrible feeling of not feeling loved.

But as the calling from God was becoming clearer to me, I knew I needed to change my attitude. In 1994, in Pittsburgh, I learned the value of a vision and a game plan. My first baseball hero, the late Roberto Clemente, was being honored in the All-Star game which was in Pittsburgh that year. It occurred to me how wonderful it would be to be able to create sports memorabilia honoring him. I knew about needing an artist to put the products together, but I didn't realize that there were licensing fees for the Clemente family, the Pirates, and Major League Baseball Organization. I found it was going to cost $30,000! I didn't have any resources for all of that! So, I put together a presentation and started reaching out to people who could be investors. I had a lot of "no" responses, but I met a kind man who believed in what I was trying to do. He listened to me, he developed a shared vision, and this little white man wrote me--a Black man in my 30s--a check for $30,000 to help me reach my goal. With his investment, I was able to commission an original painting "A Celebration of Roberto" and a series of limited edition lithographs.

After my accident and as the years passed, I was determined to return to work. So, I put in an application for a state job and became an intake worker for State Unemployment and eventually got promoted as a case worker for the Welfare Department. I gradually came to realize that I had to change my attitude and build links as I moved closer to the work God was calling me to do. I answered the call to ministry, and began the process of becoming credentialed. I became involved with several ministries, including the prison and jail ministry. By this time, I knew God was calling me to pastoral ministry. The high point of that realization came in the early 2000s and my life began to change dramatically. So this call to pastoring, had meant that I had retired from my other career in social work and that I was entering a new phase in life where I wasn't financially secure. I knew I had to trust God, be obedient and remember that God has made, and God will always make a way for us.

In 2013, I was called to pastor a church in Arizona. They were a white, very conservative congregation, completely different from the church I pastor now. Little by little, we developed personal relationships that I will always be happy to have had. Their messages to me when I headed east to pastor the Kirby Avenue Church of God in Muncie helped me to know that they loved me and appreciated the time when I was their pastor.

Marriage was never in the cards for me. (I joke that I have played hard to get for so long that it backfired on me!) Truth is, I was never really ready. Although I did have the opportunity to be a sort of father figure to others from time to time. One relationship built several years back really stands out to me now. I had the joy to work with a young man who was a distant cousin. His life was going nowhere. He had no ambitions, no goals. I helped this young man learn and, over time, discover that every person needs to be a person of character and integrity. Every person needs to have a vision for his life and a game plan on how to reach the vision. I even helped him realize he needed to build a portfolio and collect letters of reference from people with whom he had relationships with. He put his tools together and used them to get into college, and also eventually ended up getting a master's degree. He is in Pennsylvania now and has used his exercise physiology degree to start a wellness business. I cherish a letter he gave me thanking me for being a mentor in his life.

We all need to work at being mentors to someone else. Giving benefits in that way is among life's greatest blessings.

So today, I'm in Muncie. Friends from other times in my life questioned whether Muncie was going to be a good place to be. And it's the greatest! I have been here five years, and Muncie is definitely my home. I pastor a wonderful church. I've been blessed to play community roles on community boards and in organizations such as the Police Merit Board, MITS, Christian Ministries, and Muncie Neighborhood Association. I've met wonderful Christian brothers in a weekly prayer group. Building and maintaining relationships with brothers who are from several ethnicities, denominations and all walks of life have blessed me in a powerful way. We are twenty years into the 21st century. I'm headed toward my senior years and plan to keep going and serving and building relationships for years to come.

Right now, across this nation, we all need to work on our developing and strengthening of relationships, and learn from each other as our country and our world falls into deeper and deeper division. For those of us who believe that Satan gets a "foothold" (as I do), we as Christians need to facilitate turning Satan's foothold into God's stronghold. Micah 6:8 says, "He has shown you, O mortal, what is good. And what does the Lord require of you? To act justly and to love mercy and to walk humbly with your God."

The relationship I so longed to have with an earthly father in my youth never materialized. I could have let it be all consuming to a point where my life would have headed in a totally different direction. But God's mercy, my listening to His calling, and the joy of having developed links with people of varying beliefs and perspectives will sustain me. It will sustain me for the rest of my life as I continue to build relationships with others that God continues to place in my path.

Chapter 2: A Timeless Classic

Jeff Ross's Story as told to J.R. Jamison by his mother, Ann Marie Ross

CHEV - RO - LET

Lined up on the magnetic spelling board in primary colored letters. He couldn't say it, but there he was—spelling it.

CHEV - RO - LET

He was three at the time. Must've been something on television and he was relaying the message back to us. He didn't actually talk until he was four, but, you know, he's unusual. He's been to different diagnostic places, and everyone says they've never seen a case like him.

There on the old, metal magnetic spelling board –

CHEV - RO - LET

These simple, classic spelling board games . . . they really helped us when sound wasn't the determining factor to let our minds know what he was thinking.

***

Well, when Jeff was born the cord was around his neck. Which cut off oxygen, and that caused the brain damage. It wasn't obvious in the beginning, but around 11-months-old he didn't really show any signs of crawling or walking. We kind of suspected something, and when he was about 15-months-old the pediatrician confirmed that brain damage had likely occurred during birth.

But, like I say, he's an interesting case.

Jeff started reading and spelling before the age of when most children exhibit these types of developments. His speech wasn't coming along well, but he loved to read. Books on presidents, books on travel, and in kindergarten, he read an entire encyclopedia. Once his speech came, he could tell you the name of every president's wife, her birthdate—he could even tell you their anniversaries!

It was almost like he had a photographic memory.

One of his pre-school teachers at Isanogel even said, "Send him to Burris."

Burris, at the time, had four teachers per classroom because students from Ball State would go over and help the main teachers with their classes. When we'd go to parent-teacher conferences they'd say, "He just amazes the college kids."

They'd give a test, and he'd go down every question and check, check, check and be done, and everyone else was still taking it. This one girl said she thought Jeff had just marked anything to finish and that he likely didn't have any of the answers correct. So she pulled his test and checked it before the other kids got done, and every answer was right. It's like he was this little genius.

But by the time he got into middle school, he couldn't do the math.

One of his diagnoses is that the left and right side of his brain don't work together. For reading you only need one side of your brain, and for math and reasoning you need the other. And a typical brain transfers information back and forth, but, with Jeff's, only one side works at a time and doesn't connect.

Since Burris wasn't going to work out, we explored other options.

We even tried a school in Piqua, Ohio.

But after two years it became too much. We brought him back to Muncie and he went to Wilson, and then on to Southside. In 1990 he got his graduation certificate and he went over to Hillcroft to work in their workshop.

He loves it over there. He does piece work, mainly. It's repetitive.

He likes things to stay the same.

He likes to play supervisor.

During breaks, he has to be the last one to leave the lunch room so he can make sure everyone is out. And if they're not? Well, he gets a bit supervisory on them.

But that's Jeff, you know.

He'll be there until retirement. It's not like a factory, it's a good environment. When we're on vacation he says he can't wait to get back to work. We laugh and say, "Who wants to go back to work when they're on vacation?"

Hillcroft takes good care of him. I feel good about it—he's safe over there. And like I say, he doesn't communicate well.

Every now and then we do get approached about him having a job out in the community, but his sense of reasoning is just so bad. I really hesitate to do that. Like, if I told him in the morning to go down the hill to get the bus, and if the bus didn't come until 5:00 in the afternoon he'd still be sitting there. He wouldn't think, "Gee, maybe the bus isn't coming."

He has a form of aphasia.

Sometimes he'll blurt out a sentence and it's clear as can be, and other times it takes him five minutes to spit out a sentence. Between that and his lack of reasoning ability, he can't work out in public.

Even with family, the communication can be different. He does this special handshake with his nieces, where he puts his finger out and they touch it, and then he goes on and goes away. And then they do it again before they leave. And if they forget to do it, he'll stand down at the bottom of the hill and wait for them to come back.

***

Growing up, some kids would make fun of him and your heart just breaks when you see it. That's life I guess, but that was the difficult aspect of it all . . . the most challenging part of having a son with disabilities. He didn't always notice people were picking on him or being mean. Only once or twice. And when he was little, he'd cry.

But after that, it didn't seem to bother him as much.

As he's gotten older, the world has grown up around him, and Jeff has stayed so young at heart. In many ways, he's a classic case of someone with intellectual disabilities, but in other ways—such as his impeccable memory—he's not.

He's different.

He's timeless and ageless. He still sees the world as a child in many ways, and there is something really beautiful about that.

Chapter 3: Where I'm Supposed to Be

John Charles Peterson's story as told to Jeffrey Owen Pearson

Here I am, rambling away, and you, letting me tell stories. That could be the biggest mistake ever. Actually, I've written a book already, *The True Adventures of Captain Wa Wah*, where I relate my early days as a keyboard player in a band from Iowa that played gigs from Chicago to Denver, then my transition to becoming a Family Practice doctor in Muncie, Indiana.

I have no intention of retiring soon because I like what I do. What keeps me going? I've never known, not since I started 72 years ago. First, there was the musician. Then, the doctor. What I do in medicine and music, and everything else I do, is a part of my dharma...doing that which I should be doing to be happy and fulfilled. I've been fortunate enough through the years to do things that are in keeping with my dharma.

I've always been the one that was a little different. Long hair to my waist in those early years, antiwar, anti-Viet Nam, and anti-corporate.

I said to my med school, "You need someone like me here," and they said, maybe so. I'm not part of the local health conglomerate here, and I see fewer patients than other doctors. That way I get to spend more time with my patients, who are people and not numbers. The only day I didn't have a full caseload was my first day in practice, and I attract patients who are well informed. I still play music around town, and between clients I compose music in my head. I can't turn it off. Before I die, I have 40 or 50 songs I want to record. This year I will release an album with five original songs and five songs written by two iconic Hoosier composers, Hoagie Carmichael and Cole Porter.

For a number of years, I owned Doc's Music Hall in downtown Muncie. When we closed the club, the documentarian Robert Mugge asked, "Are you still a musician first?" I'll tell you what I told him. I think they're the same dharma, medicine and music. There's the same synaptic processing, synergistic patterning, and creative mathematics. Parts of the same thing.

There was a young keyboard player I taught to play. Despite his failing year after year in math, he was a masterful mathematician on the keyboard. I taught him how mathematical patterns correlate with chords. Tricks of chord progressions that give emotional experience. These were all things I figured out mathematically, combinations that trigger different emotions. Suspended chords, minors and majors. Where you play on the keyboard always makes a difference. For instance, the mus-ic of Brahms had a prominent low end. The tones themselves vibrate, much like celestial bodies.

After nearly fifty years of practice, I have all sorts of medical stories to tell. That's my next book. For instance, there's the case of a VA patient with a loss of all feeling from the waist down. I was a third-year med student in neurology rotation, and I was the one chosen to present the case to one of the world's authorities in the field. Intrigued, he took us all and went over to the VA to see the patient himself. After thoroughly examining the man I said, "I have no idea what's wrong." The lesson? Admit what we don't know, what we can't explain.

I found that by studying ancient Ayurvedic writings, I could learn time-tested wisdom. The understanding of scholars from thousands of years ago now coincides with discoveries of quantum physicists who have explained the unified field Einstein was searching for. We are basically all different frequencies, and medicine can find healing at the fundamental source of our existence.

I had a patient with ITP, a disease where the body forms antibodies against its own blood cells called platelets. Basically, the body is at war with itself. The regimen we tried, based on Vedic knowledge, was successful, and she later chaired a symposium on the disease and asked me to represent an alternative medical viewpoint. I asked a Vedic scholar and physician for advice. After much discussion, he noted that autoimmune issues are all indicators of unexpressed anger. Remember, he told me, the most important thing is healing. Practice unconditional forgiveness.

I feel really fortunate. My wife, Vicki, is wonderful. The kids and grandkids are great, and this Christmas was a joy spending time with them. It was exhausting, but fun. It was filled with some really good and insightful conversations too. I have great friends, great patients. Lathay Pegues plays drums with me, and at some point in every gig, about half way through, something happens that's unexpected and magical. I look at Lathay and say, "You know something?" and he says, "I know, Doc. It doesn't get better than this."

And that's the running joke. Whether there's two people or a hundred people in the audience. It doesn't matter. "You know something, Lathay? It doesn't get better than this."

CHAPTER 4: I'M BUSY RETIRING—PLEASE LEAVE A MESSAGE!

M. KAY STICKLE'S STORY AS TOLD TO JULIE DAVIS

Eighty percent of General Motors' lost rail cars ended up in Muncie, Indiana. It's true! And believe it or not, I did too.

In high school, I worked for General Motors in Pontiac, Michigan, so I could earn money to go to school. I worked for the parts engineering department, and in an era that made no use of computers, was assigned the task of finding all the rail cars loaded with General Motors parts that had become lost in transit. Rail cars numbered with chalk on their sides. In winter. In Michigan.

Does that sound like a challenging task? Good, because I love those! I took them on not only at General Motors, but in my undergrad work at Eastern Michigan and my graduate work at Michigan State. And when the president at Michigan State asked me to contact John

R. Emens about a job at Ball State University, I knew exactly where Muncie was.

By the time I joined the faculty at Ball State in 1968, I'd already set up 75 model reading clinics across Michigan, promoted education on the ground in dictator-led Nicaragua, and trained African-Americans to pass their Voter Literacy Test in Selma, Alabama. As a professor in the field of education, I coached teachers who would go on to invest their lives in students around the nation.

During my career, I received job offers from several places, including the University of Tennessee, Pittsburgh, and Peabody College. But although I visited each location and considered carefully whether I should move, it was always clear that Muncie was still the place for me to be. I wanted to live in the same city where I taught and invested in that community in meaningful, and long-term ways. I wanted to do what I loved.

And I didn't want to wait!

The passions and gifts I had already cultivated could be transplanted into the life of the community where I lived, worked, and worshiped. I wanted to find out where the needs were and begin to address them. When I discovered that Ball Memorial Hospital gave booties and hats to newborns, I contacted them and showed them the knitting and crochet work I could offer. They were pleased with that, and I began making baby hats and booties at home in the evenings after my workday at Ball State. Since I was still working, Sandra Hoover, the director of Volunteer Services, would call me if there was a bad winter storm. She knew I'd been willing to stop at the hospital on my way home from work and deliver flowers and cards to patients so other volunteers wouldn't have to drive in poor weather.

I planned for early retirement and took that in 2001. I wanted to be able to play—to travel at any time I wanted. But more importantly, I wanted to be busy with a purpose. I knew I needed to be active in later life just as I had earlier. And I wanted to give in the areas that pulled at my heart.

Still, I was a bit taken aback when my friend Susan Beatty, who was head of the newly reorganized Emergency Department at Ball Memorial, called and asked me to help her. "I don't want to be tied down," I said. "I retired so I could play!"

"Just come help us for a few days," she pleaded.

I protested that I didn't have a jacket. A badge. Any training. She said, "We'll get you everything you need and train you this afternoon." And that's when the adventure really began.

I fell in love.

I fell in love with the emergency department staff and the job they were doing. I loved helping patients feel comfortable and reassured. When they opened the NICU a year or so later, I loved comforting and cuddling the premature babies.

In my early fifties, I'd been surprised by a diagnosis of ovarian cancer. With the wonderful support of family and friends, I faced surgery and chemotherapy, regained my energy and stamina, and returned to work. I remember those days . . . how I hadn't known a single person who had lived through cancer, how I wondered if it would be worth it to undergo the rigorous treatment. Surely there was a way I could put that experience to use now.

And there was. The Cancer Center welcomed me with open arms, and how I loved that too! I pass out warm blankets, make hot chocolate, and simply be present as a friend to those going through treatment. Do they need encouragement? I can provide that. How about a bit of gentle, teasing fun? Also in my toolkit. And sometimes what they most need is just to tease me when I make a mistake or forget a request.

My imperfect service offers them the chance to help me remember or succeed, so that I am able to function as more of a peer for them.

Perhaps that's one of the most surprising things about giving myself to others: whether I'm volunteering in the hospital, speaking at churches or community groups, training college students, or any of the myriad things that fill my days, my willingness to give of myself returns a full blessing to me. I began singing with Survivor Voices, the chorus founded by Dr. Michael and Laura Williamson, so that I could promote hope and encouragement to cancer patients and their caregivers, but actually I too reap the benefits. I started to help Muncie Civic Theater by promoting season ticket sales and greeting guests as they arrive for performances, but it turned out I always walked away invigorated and refreshed. I grab each new adventure—knowing I may make mistakes but am willing to learn as I go—and in the end, I am filled. I am energized. And I have the joy of knowing I get to help build into my community.

I've always said I like being the legs! Don't make me the chair of something. Don't make me the president. Because I like figuring out how to get things done. Right now I'm in the midst of the shutdown for COVID-19. I can't go into the hospital, the community theater, or even my own church building. So instead, I bought a smartphone—my first! And I'm getting things done that way. I have faith that there are still good tomorrows out there, and I want to take care of myself now, stay connected now, so that as soon as restrictions are lifted, I can jump with both feet into all the ways I help build my community—and all the ways my community helps build me.

Chapter 5: The Unforgettable Now

Jerrold Thomas's Story as Told to Kelsey Timmerman

You can call me sexy.

That's what I told Miranda the first time she met me. Then she gave me water, and asked if it was cold enough. I told her it tasted like gin.

I like to say funny stuff to staff members like Miranda and my co-workers. I try to keep a straight face, but my grin always gives me away.

When I talk on the phone with my girlfriend, Debbie, she tells me I'm beautiful.

I guess I'm doing something right. My cousin, Charles, says I'm a hound dog.

What kind of guy am I? I'm a good-looking guy, like my dad. Sometimes when I look in a mirror, I see him. Dad was a heck of a baseball player. He pitched. They called him Lefty. He was a big guy. He needed to be. He was an international union organizer and worked with Walter Reuther, a former president of the UAW who survived several assassination attempts.

Dad fought for what he believed in. He was a tough guy, except with me. I was his soft spot. He taught me to drive a tractor. I drove the tractor all the time working the land, mowing the grass.

School was okay, but I'd rather have been driving through the fields. I like to move. I like to go places. I don't like to sit still. There's too much to see, too many people to meet.

My parents took me everywhere.

We drove to California on Route 66 with Charles's family. Staring out the window, I could name the make, model, and year of every car we passed. It's kind of like a superpower, I guess. I still can do it some.

I was never allowed to drive on the road, but I've always loved cars. I've got a picture of a Mustang on my wall in my room.

Charles tells me that I picked on him all the way to California and back. I remember standing on the edge of the Grand Canyon. I remember the wind, and thinking I was going to fall in. I scared the dickens out of my family.

There are a lot of moments I don't remember though. I wish that I could remember more about my mom. She was nice, really smart, and never swore. She never drank. She was a good teacher.

Dad on the other hand . . . when I turned 21, he got me drunk. I definitely don't remember much about that night. Dad would always take me to the bar with him. He was a Delaware county commissioner and he had a lot of meetings there.

Mom and Dad took me to Hawaii. I saw some Hula dancers. Even today, I can't say "hula dancers" without wiggling my eyebrows.

People loved my parents. I loved my parents.

My parents have been gone a long time. When they were here, they visited a lot. They were proud of me. I still visit them at the cemetery. I miss them, especially during the holidays. Someday I'll be next to my Mom and Dad again.

***

Last Friday my roommates and I met Debbie at KFC. It was a hot date, yup!

I tried to play it cool. I ordered my three-piece chicken meal. Got my drink, and then spilled it all over the table. Miranda said it was okay. We switched tables.

Debbie works at Hillcroft, too. I love to work, especially with her. I'm not going to say how old she is.

...Okay, if you really want to know . . . she is 30. Yup, there's an age difference between us, but who gives a heck.

We first started dating in Florida, or was it the Bahamas?

Debbie says that we've only been dating a few weeks. What does time matter? We're not sure where we went in Florida. We think it was a beach. I know I felt happy.

Some days at work we recycle CDs. Today we stuffed marketing envelopes for a local photographer. The outside of the envelopes read: "Unforgettable Moments Preserved Forever."

***

At KFC Debbie sat at the table next to me and introduced herself as my girlfriend to a new friend who joined us for dinner . . . it's not easy to eat fried chicken while smiling.

I had trouble thinking of what to talk to her about, so I said, "Debbie, are you eating a cookie?" I batted my eyes at her and she laughed.

Someone asked her what we talked about on the phone every night. This was too much. I'm kind of shy.

"More Pepsi, Debbie?" I asked.

I went to get her a refill. My sixty-seven-year old knees have arthritis, but my thirty-year-old girlfriend needed a refill, and I needed an excuse to escape that embarrassing conversation.

When I got back I posed for a picture with Debbie. That means I got to scooch over right beside her.

When it was time to go home, I said, "Bye, Debbie. See you Monday, honey. Don't forget to call me tonight."

And then I went home. I have fun at the house with my roommates and the staff. I love it . . . every minute of it.

***

I've hit home runs just like my dad. I like the Colts and the Reds, cars and cruising music. I love my cat Lovie. I've shaken the hand of the mayor and sold paintings of horses. I drink one O'Doul's a day. It's the best beer because you can take your medicine with it.

I think I'm living a good life. I'm having fun so far. The secret to living a good life and having fun is getting out and doing things.

I've had a lot of unforgettable moments. I know that. I know I felt happy in the Bahamas. I know that I enjoyed working at Bob Evans, Wendy's, and the Radisson, but sacking groceries for people at Ross's made me the happiest.

I don't remember many of the details, but remember how I felt: I've always felt loved.

My favorite unforgettable moment is now, and I feel great.

CHAPTER 6: FREEING THE SURVIVOR

LYLANNE MUSSELMAN'S STORY AS TOLD TO JACKIE HARRIS

At 63, people may look at me and think: she's doing great, she's probably had a lot of good breaks in her life. She's successful with her art, her writing, and she's still teaching classes. She looks happy. I would tell them they are right about a few of those things. However, the adage you can't judge a book by its cover is true. I have not had an easy life.

My parent's relationship had a definite effect on me. My dad was a silent and remote person throughout my life. My mom never had my best interests at heart. She used to put me in the middle of how she felt about dad and his "silent treatments." Mom was controlling, and as I've grown to learn, narcissistic. She has appeared in many of my poems and stories. Recently, I served as her caregiver and in that role, she still always wanted me with her, which was beyond my comfort level. Being in the same room with her always, when there was no reason; all I wanted to do was go to my room and write or read – it explained a lot about my parent's relationship. I feel my mom was more afraid of being alone than of being in a marriage that didn't make her happy. Besides gaining insights into my parent's relationship dynamic for the two years I was her caregiver, I also have written a lot about her dementia. In fact, I was recently nominated for a Pushcart Prize for a poem I wrote about being my mom's caregiver.

With that said, I've been in many relationships throughout my life. I married my first husband when I was 18. My two daughters are from that marriage, and they are the lights of my life. He was mentally abusive, so I was a single mom for most of their growing up, with a few other relationships and marriages tossed in. Unfortunately though, those relationships were abusive as well, mentally and physically. Nevertheless, I learned from those experiences and moved forward. Now, the security that carries me comes from my poetry, art, my family, friends, and my kitties.

Along the way, I was inspired by Natalie Goldberg's *Writing Down the Bones: Freeing the Writer Within*. This prompted me to reenroll at Ball State after dropping out 20 years earlier. Once in college, I put off taking an English class because I still thought I was a horrid writer. My initial major was graphic design. When I finally enrolled in my first English class, I had an instructor who helped me relax with writing. My subsequent teacher marked my paper up and I started doubting myself again. However, this time I was more mature. And instead of bailing college again, I talked to her and received encouragement. The more I wrote and studied English, the more I improved. I had many opportunities at Ball State, and got my poetry published while there, and my one-act play produced. Since graduating with my English degree, I've had six more one-act plays produced and I'm a widely-published poet. I have many chapbooks and books published of my poems as well. I went on to get my master's degree at University of Indianapolis, and I've been teaching writing classes of all stripes as an adjunct prof for Ivy Tech Community College for 14 years, and many other institutions as I've made my way.

I have surprised myself (and others) by putting myself in front of people – in classrooms and at poetry readings. The timid person I once was now enjoys these things.

During the rough years, there was a time when I turned my back on God and was angry that life was not kind. But I missed church, and began paying attention to friends still in the church community. I realized that my church friends had given me good advice in the past, so I turned to them again. Through them, I realized the abuse hadn't been my fault; I was the victim and I hadn't deserved the treatment I received (yes, I am one of the #MeToo victims...beginning at 15 years old). Instead of running further from God and hiding the multiple abuses, I take solace now in finding a church home and in finding my voice: I'm a survivor!

I still have some frustrations, such as money worries. I don't have much income, since I'm an adjunct instructor and an artist. Unpredictable or unexpected financial situations are difficult. Another concern is that I only have one good eye, as I was born with a birth defect. As I've aged, I've worried about going blind (not being able to draw, drive, etc.). Stubborn as I am, I don't want to lose my independence.

Through it all, finally, I'm happy with who I am. I often wonder how I didn't grow into more insecurities instead of growing out of them. I feel that credit goes to my grandma, who I was extremely close to, to my love of reading, where I gained empathy; to my natural enjoyment of solitude which is so important for my creativity, and to the teachers and professors that made a big impact on me, giving me encouragement. My high school art teacher, Ann Johnson, still to this day is my biggest cheerleader.

Retirement is not appealing for those of us in the arts. There are many cases of people being very creative in older age such as Grandma Moses and Ruth Stone. So, as I look to the future, I would like to keep my good health. Without that, everything else is a moot point. I want to keep writing, painting, and teaching. I plan to keep participating in community organizations; basically, I want to be a good creative citizen.

Both of my daughters are in healthy marriages and I enjoy my grandchildren and great-grandchildren. I am happy that through all my daughters saw me go through, they learned what not to do. They have better marriages than I thought possible. They give me hope!

Chapter 7: A Life Coach Full of Surprise

Rodelyn McPherson's Story as Told to Jackie Harris

I had the privilege and blessing to be born and raised in sunny Southern California before smog and overcrowding. The ocean was close by, the mountains visible, and the desert not far; all easily accessible. Daily, I could count on a lovely breeze that began around 4 p.m. I never heard the term "rain date," as the sunshine was as reliable as the breeze.

I was gifted with a joyful spirit, enthusiasm, optimism, an overdeveloped sense of humor, leadership skills, athletic abilities, acting chops, and excellent health. Of course though, I didn't know this right away. But I knew early that I was curious, loved discovery, and had a sense of awe and wonder. All these God given talents developed, grew and flourished beginning in junior high and through high school and led to many experiences that could fill a book. On the downside, if I wasn't good at something in a week, I would quit trying. My poor parents were patient, as I went through every musical instrument known to man.

There was an interval after high school and during college when my idyllic life changed sharply. I married very young and soon realized I was in a harsh and very verbally-abusive relationship. This was a major learning experience that taught me that not everyone lives as I had lived. I was aware that my natural born gifts seemed to die. My self-esteem was less than zero. I seriously considered maybe I should die.

The relationship ended as I graduated from college and began teaching elementary school. At night, I was heavily involved in theatre. Which eventually led to my being asked to go to New York to do theatre.

In 1962, I took a Greyhound Bus and wended my way through the southern states making stops along the way to visit cities. In Baton Rouge, I saw prejudice and bigotry as I could have never imagined. While in Miami, during the Cuban influx of refugees, as Castro let them leave, Floridians were at the docks not yelling "welcome," but things like "I need a gardener, housekeeper, nanny, cook, driver," etc. as if there weren't any doctors, lawyers or professors among them. After two weeks, I arrived in Muncie to visit my sister and her husband, who was the football coach at Taylor University. And I have been in this area ever since. The show I was invited to be in never "hit the boards" as it was scheduled to open the week of President Kennedy's assassination.

Later at age 35, with a husband and 4 kids, I realized that I had to honor these God given gifts by nurturing, using (use it or lose it), and sharing them to serve God and others. When my children were ages 1, 2, and 3, I had an apron that read, "For this I spent 7 years in college?" and a huge poster in my kitchen that had a toddler with a bowl of spaghetti on his head with the contents running down his face and it read, "This is the Day that the Lord has made. I Will Rejoice and be Glad in it." Yay! Sense of humor!

I have been aware of God's presence in my life since I was 15 years old; not that I walked the straight and narrow since then. I wrestled with doubt, questions and such after witnessing some very ugly expressions of Christianity.

But at 35, I asked God to be my life coach. God opened the door to summer softball coaching of high school girls, long-term substitute teaching jobs, and many volunteer opportunities such as the chairperson of book fairs, a librarian, and plenty of coaching positions. But the greatest opportunity was being a stay-at-home mom.

The only time I cried till I sobbed was when I realized I would be 50 when my youngest child graduated high school...Sob...I'll be so old. But at 50, I began the career of my life.

WARNING: God's life coaching is full of surprises.

I became a minister, and was the Lutheran Campus Minister at Ball State for 20 years. "Take that age 50!" What a privilege, blessing, and an opportunity to use all my God given gifts!

I retired from Campus Ministry, but not ministry. Thankfully, I'm still using my gifts at my church and other churches. Among other activities, I'm an Adult Christian Education Facilitator. Another valuable use of my time is that I volunteer at Ball Hospital every Thursday in the ICU and the Library of Life, Love and Laughter. Additionally, I'm also a member of 3rd Age Theatre, an entertainment group.

People think I'm so busy, but believe me, I have plenty of down time (as in days when I don't have activities or expectations). Every day I do a short stretching and exercise routine. I spend anywhere from a half hour to an hour just sitting and praying in God's presence and expressing how I'm so grateful for the way I've been blessed.

Recently, I read that the happiest people have three things in common: exercise, meditation, and gratitude. At 81 ½, I'd say, "I nailed it!"

Thanks once again to God, my life coach.

CHAPTER 8: FACING RACISM WITH HELP

SAM ABRAM'S STORY AS TOLD TO LAUREN BISHOP-WEIDNER

My father, Lonnie Abram, was the most efficient picker on the Money, Mississippi, cotton plantation where he sharecropped, a distinction that earned him $1.00 each week as well as permission to travel to Greenwood and to cut hair on weekends. In 1940s Mississippi, a person of color still needed permission from a plantation owner just to be on the roads. My father was valuable enough to the landowner that he was given the privilege to travel as well as to earn a little extra money barbering. A car accident left him with an injured right hand, poorly cared for in an outbuilding behind the hospital. As a result of the injury, he couldn't pick cotton or use the barber chair on the street outside a business owned by a relative of the landowner.

We moved to Muncie in 1944, staying with relatives until he got a job and could buy a house. Although my mother stayed in Mississippi, my father never let us lose touch with her. My father drove the nearly 1400-mile round trip in a weekend, making sure we got to Memphis by 6:00 a.m. in order to buy gas—any later, and we might not be served.

Once we hit the Mississippi line, his caution increased greatly—remember, Emmett Till was murdered in Money, Mississippi. We'd head back to Muncie in time for my father to be ready for work at 6:00 a.m. Monday. From a very early age, I saw the sacrifices my father made for his family.

Leroy Ash, a neighbor several years older than I, was like a big brother. He helped with homework and encouraged me to try new things. Kids from Mississippi didn't just automatically fit in. We looked different, we sounded different. Some of the local boys took advantage, but Mr. Ash helped me to gain the confidence I needed. He worked at the Branch YMCA on Madison Street, and I'd go there after school. When I was new to softball, I wasn't a very good hitter. After two strikes, someone would usually beg for my last strike. Seeing this, Mr. Ash asked me:

"How many strikes do you get?"

"Three," I answered.

"And how many are you taking?"

"Two."

"Sam, you can't give away the opportunities you're given."

That advice stayed with me all my life.

I used to follow Mr. Ash around the Y, helping out wherever I could. When I was a little older, I applied for a job there. Mr. Roy Buley, Director of the Branch YMCA, hired me because he'd seen me helping out and he trusted Mr. Ash's recommendation.

In the mid-1950s, the city planned a new building for the Madison Street YMCA, but it was to remain a segregated facility. Many in the neighborhood were overjoyed, but not Mr. Buley. Well known and highly respected, he'd walk through the community talking with people. He included me in these conversations, as he explained that we needed to desegregate the downtown Y if we were going to have equal access to facilities and programs. Mr. Buley's logic escaped most, and plans for the new building came to pass. History proved Mr. Buley to be right. I was privileged to learn from his example of courage, dignity, and leadership.

My first dream was to be an Air Force pilot, the result of stories I heard from one of my elementary teachers, Mr. Dygert, who had been a fighter pilot and a real hero. I enrolled in Ball State's ROTC program, majoring in Social Studies, Driver's Education, and Business. Halfway through my junior year, I passed everything I needed to in order to continue—except for the eye exam. I needed a new goal. With my major, high school teaching would have been a logical path. Unfortunately, Muncie was not hiring high school teachers who were Black, and I didn't want to leave Muncie. At that time, Muncie had five Black teachers, all at one or the other of the two Longfellow Elementary buildings. After petitioning to take a double overload in order to complete the necessary credit hours for an Elementary Education license, I graduated on time.

I was deeply committed to learning as much as I could during my student teaching at West Longfellow. I typed my lesson plans and organized my materials carefully, hoping my efforts would lead to a job offer for the following school year. I knew if I wasn't hired at Longfellow, I wouldn't have a teaching job—no other school in Muncie would have even considered my application. Mr. Burl Clark was principal, and we met twice that spring. The second time, he told me that he wasn't going to recommend me because he was pushing for schools other than Longfellow to open up for teachers of color. Thanks to Mr. Clark, Doris Faulkner transferred from Longfellow to become the first African-American teacher in Blaine School, and I began that fall of 1960 teaching fifth grade at East Longfellow.

While teaching, I continued my education and in 1966 became principal at Longfellow, a job I cherished for four years. When I wanted to transfer to a larger school, I was told I would not be transferred, and not to ask again. The excuse given was that I was the youngest elementary principal. The truth was that I was Black. I looked for a new job. I accepted an excellent upper administration position with Marion Community Schools and tendered my resignation.

Then I got a phone call on a Sunday evening from Dr. Robert Freeman, who had been hired that weekend as Superintendent of Muncie Community Schools. I was abrupt with him, telling him I already had a job. He was patient with me, explaining that he wouldn't have called me if he hadn't already spoken with the Marion Superintendent. I accepted the position he offered as his Administrative Assistant, and he continued to mentor me, modeling and teaching necessary skills. After three years, I took a leave of absence to complete my doctorate, and in 1989 I became Superintendent of Muncie Community Schools.

God has blessed me with many mentors, and my path grew clear as I learned from every one of them. My father, Mr. Ash, Mr. Buley, Mr. Dygert, Mr. Clark, Dr. Freeman, and so many others, Black and White—without their leadership and guidance, I would not have become the man God intended me to be. I pray that God has used me in the same way, to help shape the lives of others.

CHAPTER 9: THE 11TH MOST WANTED MAN IN AMERICA

ALLEN F JOHNSTONE'S STORY AS TOLD TO JAMES E MITCHELL

I'm Australian, so I hope you can come waltz the matilda with me as I tell you about my newest project.

In October 2019, I agreed to join the board of the Muncie/Delaware County Senior Citizens Center. I've always believed that we should use whatever skills and experiences we have to change things.

How did an Aussie find himself in the States, and in Muncie, Indiana, you might wonder?

I arrived for a visit in New York the same year that another Aussie made his home there. (You might recall Mike from the film "Crocodile" Dundee II?) The year was 1989 and I was the CEO of UNICEF Queensland, based in Brisbane, Australia. I was called over here to give a paper at the United Nations.

Before I returned to Brisbane, I stayed at a hotel outside the city and noticed it had 13 floors. I took the lift to the 12th floor and 13th floor, and both had steel doors and cameras but no markings. I asked at reception what was happening on those floors and found out it was the local headquarters of the FBI. Immediately, I asked the hotel clerk to ring the FBI and ask him if I could take a tour. He agreed. I got a tour just by asking, including the wall with the Ten Most Wanted List photographs. To prove I had been there, I had my picture taken next to the other usual suspects. Does that make me the Eleventh Most Wanted Man in America?

After taking my family on a world tour, I returned to the States in 1991 and have been here since. My brother and sister lived in Los Angeles for years before retiring to East Central Indiana near Fairmount. I have a history of starting businesses, including the Australian Museum of Muncie and Anderson, a jewelry store, a restaurant, and a banquet room. I even had a stint working on creating a themed attraction in New Jersey.

Now, the Muncie/Delaware County Senior Citizen Center is the place where I invest my time, talent, experience, and connections.

I first visited the center with my wife for lunch during the senior cafe. After our meal, someone approached us and asked if I would be willing to serve on the board of the organization. I was already serving with the wonderful people at Open Door Health Services, where my wife volunteered me. As I considered the question, and before I could open my mouth to respond, I heard a "yes" -- it came not from me, but from my side: my wife spoke up and agreed for me (again).

I had no experience with these types of centers previously, but as a businessman and media professional, I knew how I could learn. Before my first board meeting, I spent weeks researching best practices and American government rules to help me better understand the work of senior centers. I identified eleven changes for improvement and presented them to the board during my first meeting. I partnered with Ron, owner of a local firm, to use his marketing skills to design promotional materials. This made it easier to share my vision, and made it more likely to bring my vision to fruition.

My service as board chair started in January. I've consulted with business owners, law enforcement, and government officials one-on-one, including the mayor, to ask them for feedback and for how they can help me make this building a welcoming place that offers more programs for seniors in our area. There are tons of things going on and all of them will be supported by grants to serve the residents of the county and surrounding areas. We've been able to engage a pro bono lawyer, get technology access and printers, and we are excited to welcome guests.

We are not doing that now because of the pandemic.

COVID-19 has given us a silver lining: by being shut down, we have been able to get things done, including engaging the ingenuity of our crew to create new tables for the boardroom and create spaces for universal use. We enhanced our security measures to keep people safe from people who do not belong in the building. We are actively supporting the people we need to support through a phone bank, even in this circumstance.

Why do I do all this?

My wife considers my experience as something to benefit the community in which we live.

While it isn't my life's motto, I hung copies of a poem around the center. It is there to remind our clients they are in control of their fates, that they are "captains" of where their "ships" go. One stanza seems especially relevant to where our visitors are in life:

And yet the menace of the years
Finds and shall find me unafraid.

- Invictus by William Ernest Henley

I never pictured this is what my life would look like but I have learned to roll with the punches. I want to see change. I want to walk the talk. I don't have enough energy, not enough years left, to mess around.

Chapter 10: Facing Aging

Ron Groves's Story as Told to Donna Penticuff

My art career actually started when I was a resident of the Delaware County Children's home. Apparently, my dad wasn't happy when I became his ninth son. I think he took one look at me and left home. We lost our mother from pneumonia shortly after my fifth birthday. The County Welfare Department took me with my brothers Dick (7) and Ray (9) to the Children's Home.

When I was 11, our division was blessed with a wonderful new governess -- Mrs. Middleton. She taught us how to paint and create decorations during holidays. That's when I discovered my love for art. Two years later, my brother Dick (15) and I were taken out of the home by foster parents. Ray (now 17) was already living in another foster home. Before I left, I promised Mrs. Middleton I would become an artist when I grew up.

During my sophomore year at Yorktown High School, my foster parents offered to pay for a correspondence course in commercial art if I would give up playing basketball. It was a tough decision, but I chose the art course. I graduated from the art school the same year I received my high school diploma in 1950.

Delaware Engraving was where I began my professional career. I worked there during the summers while attending the John Heron School of Art and Design. When I was about to be drafted during the Korean War, I joined the Army. After graduating from Army Administration School at Ft. Knox, I received orders to ship out to the Far East. When the captain in charge of our group learned that I was an artist, he said they needed me to work on the ship's newspaper and pulled me off of guard duty. Fortunately, instead of going to Korea, I was one of three who was ordered off the ship in Yokohama, Japan and assigned to General Ridgeway's Headquarters in Tokyo.

After the Korean Armistice in 1953, I rented a one-room apartment in Oimachi, a small suburb north of Tokyo, where I painted portraits of wives, girlfriends, and pets for guys in my outfit.

Delaware Engraving still had my job open after my discharge in 1954 and I worked there until I was hired by the Applegate Advertising Agency. Even though I had been promoted to Art Director, I chose to leave and opened a graphic art studio in January, 1960. We became a full-service advertising agency in 1974.

My company was the collateral agency for Delco Electronics in Kokomo for 33 years. In addition to creating all the consumer literature for Delco radio sound systems and other Delco electronic products, I received an Advertising Addy Award for creating the consumer literature introducing the new "GM cell phone" in the early '90s. I also had the opportunity to create the sales' materials to promote the dual temperature controls for Buick.

I can take credit for designing the Merchants National Bank logo (...still being used), and the stylized eagle design for American National. We also worked for two divisions of Ball Corporation, Marsh Supermarkets, Westinghouse Large Power Transformers, and many others

I don't have enough space to list. We were serving up to 22 active clients during the '80s. Everything we did in those days was created using typewriters for copy, magic markers for layouts, and all printer make-ready on drawing boards.

In 1978, I opened a branch office in Fort Wayne to handle the public relations for eight Pepsi plants and served as the ad agency for the Holsum Bread Co. We had a crew of 16 people at the time – three administrative personnel in Fort Wayne, and a sales and production staff of 13 in Muncie. When Holsum Bread was sold to Bunny Bread in Lafayette, I resigned the Pepsi account and moved everything back to Muncie.

In the early '90s, I had the opportunity to work with Judge Steven Caldemeyer as he developed plans to replace the old children's home, where I was raised. I volunteered my agency to create all the fund-raising materials for the first two cottages. I didn't want to call the new facility a children's home, and asked Steve if we could use the "Youth Opportunity Center" for the name. I too, designed the logo for this center, which is still being used today.

I thought I was ready to retire in 1993. I sold my building and the furniture and equipment. After one week. I found I couldn't handle it. I called Dave Robertson, who had purchased most of my stuff, and asked him if I could have some of it back. Since he owned the White River Plaza, he said he also had available office space for me. It's hard to believe that was 27 years ago, however, most of the equipment has been replaced with computers, scanners and printers. I am at my office every weekday and sometimes working at night at home. In addition to the many clients, I was privileged to serve, you may remember the animated commercials created for the McQuik's Oilube bunny and "Mr. Blue," the blue bag recycling character for Muncie Sanitary District.

One of my most challenging projects was to create a computer-generated 10'x40' mural illustrating the history of the White River. This large vinyl print-out was hung on the wall across from the MCL Cafeteria at the Muncie Mall for a couple of years. The story was then expanded to a 9'x125' mural displayed outside at the Water Pollution Control Facility, off of Ind. 32. I have been honored to have served on the Board of Directors of the Indiana Federation of Advertising Agencies, Indianapolis, the Muncie Jaycees, the Muncie PAL Club, the Muncie Boys and Girls Club, Muncie Clean and Beautiful, and Downtown Development Partnership. In 1968, I served as Vice President of the building corporation that built the Yorktown High School on Tiger Drive and Pleasant View Elementary.

I have also worked with some great local groups such as Motivate Our Minds, the Yorktown Methodist Church, Midwest Writers Workshop, and so many others. My current project is promoting the Muncie/Delaware County Senior Citizens Center, with hopes to expand it into the adjacent former Forest Park Elementary school building. We are proposing that some of the classrooms be converted into on-site offices for a health clinic, LifeStream, local Veterans, and others associated with our seniors' well being.

The year 2020 was a big year for me – I celebrated 60 years in the advertising and graphic art business. And on July 2, 2020, I celebrated 50 years of being married to the sweetest person I know, Mary.

Mary and I love our family, enjoy traveling and are blessed to have great friends.

Thank you, Donna, for your patience and allowing me to tell my story. Maybe one of these days I will feel like I am old enough to try to retire again.

Chapter 11: I Choose to Be Happy; I Choose to Be Busy

Earlene Jeakle's Story as Told to Kathy Mulroony

Thirty-seven years ago in 1985 I married Glen Jeakle, "Jake" to his friends. He was a P-38 fighter pilot in World War II and Charles Lindberg taught him how to save fuel, a critical skill over the Pacific Ocean. His fellow pilots were like brothers when they came together for their reunions, however, their numbers dwindled and only four men attended the last event.

Glen had two children, but I never had any of my own. Now that Glen is gone, I have no family left. I sit in "widows' row" in church with my friends and I tell people that I'm an orphan!

You can make yourself as miserable as you want. I choose to be happy. It's much more satisfying that way. In fact, meeting people and entertaining large groups brought me great joy throughout my life.

My husband and I both grew up near the water, he in Detroit and I in Auburn. I studied accounting at IPFW in Fort Wayne and then I worked in the Borg Warner accounting department for 40 years, 20 of those years in Auburn, and 20 in Muncie. I was a pricing analyst with 30 interns on my staff. I believe that if you're there all day, you may as well make someone happy. And that is what I tried to do.

Glen worked in Borg Warner's engineering department where he developed some patents. Borg Warner is where we met. I saw him, got to know him, and the rest is history.

When we came to Muncie there was no question about building a pool to go with our new house. For many years, I have been swimming every day in my back yard as the weather permits. I have often cooked and hosted poolside pitch-ins with my neighbors. They keep an eye out for me, and check up on my health and safety. I love this neighborhood and consider them dear friends. We help each other and that is what dear friends do.

I love to cook and bake. Red velvet cake, pineapple upside down cake, and fruit cobblers are my favorites. I have loved entertaining over the years and have entertained 250 people in Auburn, and 70 to 80 people in Muncie, with rented chafing dishes included!

In my later years, luncheons at High Street Methodist Church have helped me stay in touch with many friends. Those, and similar outings at other venues, have kept me engaged, busy, and up to date with current events. Did I mention that I like to be busy? As long as God keeps me in good health, I plan to stay that way in my own home. It keeps me going and I just don't think about getting old.

I have traveled to Italy and Ireland, and even went on a Paris river cruise. Although the Pandemic got in the way, I planned in 2021 to join the High Street Travelers on day and overnight trips to places such as Dallas, a bluegrass celebration, and one mystery destination.

Locally, you might see me driving. Yes, driving. At 93! After all, independence makes it so much easier to stay busy!

Chapter 12: Content at 73: Diligent Worker and Vietnam Vet Battles PTSD to Find Joy

Richard Hardesty's Story as Told to Linda Marie Bicksler

Back in the mid-60s, as a young Splicer-in-training for Indiana Bell, I learned how to connect cable between high telephone poles. This initiative changed the way rural Hoosiers talked to each other forever.

Before 1967, most homes in Delaware and Madison counties operated on a Party Line. Often, 16 families (or 12, or 8) shared one line. Although they weren't supposed to, residents could hear neighbors' phone calls if they listened in (if they didn't wait for their family's special ring).

Upon graduating high school, Indiana Bell hired me and hundreds of others to connect wire for lines shared by just two or four homes. Five months in (June 1965), I became a regular Cable Splicer. But I was in Vietnam in 1967, the year that any Hoosier family who wanted a private, single-party line finally got one. Our cable made that possible.

I was drafted into the U.S. Army on May 10, 1966. (I remember exact dates, when they're important.)

After basic training in Fort Knox, Ky., and doing Army work for eight months in Fort Jackson, S.C., I had finally volunteered to go to Vietnam.

My year overseas, March 1967 to March 1968, changed me.

Yes, I was fortunate. I wasn't injured. God saw fit to keep me alive. Another blessing: I knew I'd have a good place to return to when I came back. Indiana Bell saved my job.

So I was one of the lucky ones. Yet I could never understand why I was able to come home and others couldn't.

You'd have to know what I was like to grasp how I changed.

I was 9 years old when my family moved to Gaston. I loved that small school. Everybody knew everybody, from kindergarten to 12th grade. Teachers took a special interest. My senior class, the largest ever, had 48 students.

My classmates voted me the "Wittiest." Friends nicknamed me "Big R," for Richard, like the larger-than-life character in the country song, "Big John." Students liked my joking humor. "Don't ever change," they'd say. "Stay just the way you are!"

The Vietnam Conflict affected me. I didn't realize it until much later. After returning, I became dogmatic. Bullheaded. Awfully judgmental. I had my opinion; I thought I was right. I could be a real pain in the buttocks!

Stationed in Qui Nhon (kwee non), I helped our team restore phone services to hospitals, post exchanges, mess halls, the South Vietnamese Police Department, and more.

I joke that I went to Vietnam because, first of all, I disliked "KP" (Kitchen Patrol). Vietnam was one sure way to get out of KP since Vietnamese people cooked for us. Second, I got tired of guys coming back, telling me things that were going on. Third, being overseas could mean an "early out." If you came back with three months (or less) on your Tour of Duty, you could finish early.

So I did; I served 22 months and two days in Vietnam.

That's how I deal with stress: joking around. But Vietnam grew serious. Out of the 24 guys I graduated high school with, seven went to Vietnam. Two of these, maybe more, died of Agent Orange problems.

In Qui Nhon, we always knew when our troops had faced a bad "fire night." One after another, choppers would arrive. Hospital personnel would show up at our camp, asking for certain blood types. At the three Evac hospitals nearby, we'd donate blood as often as we were allowed to.

The first dead Viet Cong I ever saw was in Summer 1967. It had a lasting impact on me. (I no longer watch fireworks on the Fourth of July.)

One evening, Viet Cong snuck into the South Vietnamese Ammunition Depot. They blew it up, all night long. On the side of a mountain, U.S. choppers kept dropping flares, launching rockets, shooting machine guns -- trying to get the VC to flee. Looked like the biggest fireworks display you've ever seen.

Next day, I walked into the depot and immediately saw a dead VC. He was lying on his back with hands and feet in the air as if he'd been crawling when he got killed. His whole body was burned black and crispy, like a marshmallow toasted too long on a campfire. It was a gruesome sight I never forgot.

My base camp was attacked three times. Our worst attack, the so-called Tet Offensives, was one of the Vietnam Conflict's major battles.

The enemy didn't always play fair. In January 1968, during the Lunar New Year, the North Vietnam government asked for a one-day truce. Its Viet Cong army used that day to move its troops and weapons into place. Seeing the explosions, Jan. 30, we first thought they were fireworks, celebrating New Year.

The next day, driving across town, we saw that the Vietnamese Police Station was all but destroyed. We kept driving; we didn't stop; but as we tried to skedaddle, the VC kept shooting -- at us. I was 21, but scared.

One memory got buried so deep, it didn't surface until a visit to the Philippines in 2018. That same Jan. 31, 1968, I stood underneath a control tower at the airfield. Suddenly a Sgt. Taylor, next to me, jerked his head to one side. "Did you hear that?" he asked me intensely.

I hadn't! My hearing was bad, a hazard of the job. Tracing a path in the sand, we came upon a lead projectile. The sergeant tried to pick it up, but couldn't keep his grip! -- it was too hot. Had either of us been standing 14 to 16 inches to his right or my left, that bullet would have blasted one of us in the head.

It took 50 years and nine months to recall that strange moment.

Another grisly event came the day the Tet Offensives stopped. Bodies in Qui Nhon had to be hauled out. These filled six trucks, each weighing "a deuce and a half" (2½ tons). Due to the holiday, men's bodies had to lie in the hot sun for days. Maggots crawled out of them. I will never forget seeing 30,000 pounds of dead enemy.

My last weeks in Vietnam, I was transferred to a new telephone office. I'd requested the change because we had all heard of the phone maintenance men who were killed outside during their last 90 days. One friend, a Sgt. Dan in the 39th SIG Battalion, came in to wish us goodbye; he was due to leave Vietnam in two days. That same night, at a USO show at the Enlisted Men's Club, someone announced on stage that the next song, Danny Boy, was dedicated to Sgt. Dan, our close buddy. Out in the valley, that afternoon, a sniper had shot and killed him. It was a very, very sad evening.

My time working indoors didn't last long; the Army needed me. I finished my Vietnam tour working outside.

I returned to Fort Lewis, Washington, in 1968. It wasn't until 2009 – more than 40 years later -- that a civilian shrink told me I had PTSD (Post Traumatic Stress Disorder).

Seeing a therapist was my pastor's idea, after I had faced a summer of family crises. My father passed away in July 2009. The day after he died, doctors had to amputate my mom's right leg above the knee. After breaking her leg, she entered a nursing home to rehabilitate it. Neglect at the facility caused gangrene. This broke my heart.

My new shrink said I needed help; he assigned me to VA care.

All the warning signs had been there for years: my dependence on alcohol, which I gave up in 1975. My four marriages. The times I contemplated suicide for over two years. (About 180,000 Vietnam Vets, I learned in 2010, committed suicide after returning home.)

Every family loss or tragedy hit me hard. My brother Dennis passed away in 2013; I lost my mom, Alma, in 2018. This left me with one family member, my sister Joyce. Being able to take care of my father's, brother's, and Mom's funeral services though, did mean something to me.

It took years to understand what happened to me in Vietnam. On the outside, I often looked okay!

During my 45 years with Indiana Bell, in all of the different positions I worked there, I only missed work two times. Both days fell during the Jan. 1978 blizzard. I came home one night to discover my jeans were solid ice, from hips to ankles. I thought I had frostbite. (Thank God I didn't.) But it did hurt when I started to get warm. That led to two days of flu.

So that winter was the end of outdoor telephone work for me.

The longest day I had ever worked outside was 40 and a half hours straight -- no break -- up on high poles, during a bad storm that tore down three cables.

Outside work, however, I struggled. The Apostle Paul said he was the "chiefest of sinners," but I don't think he beat me by much. I cussed, smoked, drank, and did many other sins -- and still thought I was a Christian. I'm not proud of who I was and the things I've done.

Today, I'm blessed to have friends who love and accept me. If I had advice to give them, it would be: "Don't wait so long to know Jesus Christ as the Lord and Savior of your life." It took me until age 29.

On Feb. 26, 1976, at a home Bible study near Commack, Ind., Pastor Myron Oiler explained what I needed to do to become a true Christian. He led me in a sinner's prayer. Two weeks later, I was baptized in the Holy Spirit -- began to sing and pray in the Spirit. I had never been to a church like that before.

The Bible says when we confess our sin, God will be faithful to forgive our sin. The Holy Spirit helped me to grow and receive forgiveness.

I've had times when I've had to swallow my pride, admit I did backslide. But when I sin, my pastor, Larry Delaney, reminds me of the Prodigal Son. That's the story where a loving Father (God) runs to greet his returning son, throws his arms around him, and holds a real blow-out party for the son who was lost, the "sinner."

These days, I like to encourage, show compassion, if I can. My favorite is the "Pentecostal Handshake," where you roll money in the hand, then, with a simple shake, pass the cash onto somebody else.

I like to tell a single Mom: "Here, why don't you take your kids and get a nice lunch. I just want to bless you."

Some days I pray for a person I see walking down a street, or inside a store. I might distribute LifeSaver mints or Gummy candy. There's the blessing of a smile, a hug, a pat on the back, a song, or an affirming word. My goal is to listen to Jesus' voice and do as he directs me.

Working part-time at Chick-Fil-A, I've so enjoyed meeting and making new friends. Although I'm retired, this is a chance to talk to a pregnant young teen or pray for an out-of-town woman battling cancer.

With good health, I've been able to see all 50 States, travel to eight countries, and enjoy four cruises. My house is paid for; my vehicle is paid for; I am blessed to "owe no man anything but to love him" (Rom. 13:8).

I've seen the joy on my daughters' and grandchildren's faces when I've been able to show up with money, give them a working vehicle, or just take them out for a big birthday bash – do something special for them.

At 73, I hope to leave fond memories, a legacy. I want my family to be able to say, "Remember Grandpa?" and "Remember Dad?"

To think back, and have a good memory.

Chapter 13: After Kazakhstan

Brenda Miller's Story as Told to Eric Miller

I have learned that life is a series of milestone events that we look back on. Which ultimately becomes the "before and after" points for us. Many tend to be relatively minor, even "normal," and then a few are major defining moments in our lives. I experienced the "normal" turning points that many people experience: moving from a very small rural town to a bigger city, going away to college, getting married, and having children. These, and others, have had a cumulative effect on my life, and have even helped shape me into the woman I have become.

I am 68 years old. I've been married to the same man, Eric, for 47 years. I have two grown sons, Matt, 46, and Andy, 40. We have two grandchildren. I am a follower of Jesus, but I'm not religious. I am an active, confident woman at this stage of my life, and accepting new challenges all the time. But the woman I am today is the result of many defining moments I had faced as a younger woman.

One defining moment came when I had to decide for whom or for what I would live my life. Having grown up in a conservative, rather judgmental church, I had learned how to avoid negative judgment by making sure I appeared "good," but I knew it was all for show. At a certain point, as a young mother, I knew I had to decide if I was going to get serious about following Jesus, or continue to go through the motions for the sake of those who might judge me. Or decide if I just wanted to give up on church altogether. So, in a time of desperate prayer, I had an experience with Jesus that showed me I no longer needed to gain the approval of any person. I was free to pursue Jesus, and live my life to please Him. This changed the trajectory of my life. I began to intentionally pursue Jesus, making knowing Him my goal. Eric, my husband, eventually joined me in that pursuit.

We decided to leave that conservative denomination that we had both grown up in, a defining moment itself, and we began attending a more "active" church. This church was active in many ways: in music worship, in meeting local needs, and in making Jesus known on a global level. We welcomed this new context of pursuing Jesus. And we were welcomed to become a part of the many ways the church was active.

We were drawn to the global activity of the church. The first major step for us as a family was to participate in a short-term fact-finding trip to Damascus, Syria. So, we somewhat nervously stepped out, took our two sons and spent three months in Damascus. This was in 1990, before the Desert Storm and that whole situation. This time was an eye-opening event for us, showing us we could step out and do something that was kind of scary.

Two-and-a-half years after we returned from Syria, we left for the newly independent country of Kazakhstan. Our new church had a vision of sending a team there, but since we were ready before they had gotten to that point, they sent us as a sort of "first fruit." Our older son, Matt, had just started college and so chose not to go with us. Leaving him and my elderly mother was the hardest thing I had done up to that point. But I was confident that Jesus would go with us, and that the prayers of our church would be fulfilled: that we would adapt quickly, make significant friendships, learn language easily, and become effective at demonstrating the life and character of Jesus to the Kazakh people.

I believe Jesus was with us, but it seemed that none of the prayers people had prayed for us came about the way they - and we - had believed they would. Life in the small town in south central Kazakhstan was hard. We found ourselves in a time warp forty or fifty years in the past. Modern conveniences were not to be had. Just finding a refrigerator took weeks, and we learned that many people didn't own one at all. Food wasn't available pre-cooked. Canned food and frozen food didn't exist in our town. The only ground beef was what I ground by hand myself. So I spent much of my time in food acquisition and preparation.

Language did not come easily. The Kazakh language was very difficult for me, being nothing like I had ever heard. They even used a completely different alphabet. My language ability did not progress much beyond that of a small child. As a result, people often spoke to me like I was a child, which was humiliating. Eric and our younger son, Andy, who was twelve-and-a-half when we first arrived seemed to have much less trouble learning than I did. As they developed meaningful friendships with Kazakh people, I felt more and more isolated.

Then, even my 43-year-old body began to betray me. My hormones began to speak a different language that I didn't recognize. I felt like I was on the edge of a cliff, with the ground under my feet increasingly unsteady. I was sure if something didn't change soon - like returning to America - I would go over the edge.

So, after only two-and-a-half years into what Eric had seen as a lifetime calling, we decided we needed to go back home. I went with much guilt, but also with a sense of relief. Eric went kicking and screaming, angry and withdrawn. I began seeing a counselor soon after we got back. Even so, ten years passed before I was able to have a right perspective of myself and of God. I hadn't failed. God had not failed.

I had obeyed what I believed God had asked of us. I had been willing to get up and leave everything behind.

"Kazakhstan" became a defining moment in my life. I could look back and see life before Kazakhstan, where after years of trying, I had come to the place of being willing to do what I believed God wanted me to do. After Kazakhstan, I came home disappointed and defeated. I had to start all over, first figuring out what I believed, throwing out almost everything except that Jesus loved me and that he had died for my sins. Before Kazakhstan, I was shallow, always wanting to be the center of attention, expecting God to make my life easy. After Kazakhstan, I came to realize that God is with me. Giving me hope, joy, and love, and giving me the strength to step out and face whatever the next defining moment in my life may be.

Now, as a woman over sixty, I have confidence to reach out and do new things. Now, I teach other older adults how to be physically fit. But I do more than teach classes. I reach out to these people who are often marginalized by society, check up on them, let them know about senior activities, and mostly try to let them know I care about them.

I have become involved with a women's addiction recovery house. I meet with the women, distribute their medicines, and have a time of Bible devotions and prayer. I go with them to different activities, like concerts or AA meetings. I even act as a supervisor when they have children visits.

I have become active in the church again, now I lead the group of ushers and greeters. I take my responsibility very seriously. I love being the one to greet people and reach out to visitors who may feel awkward or uncomfortable among people they don't know.

I am able to do all these things - and more - because I know Jesus is with me, and always giving me what I need. I no longer expect life to be easy. But I am confident that just as Jesus brought me through traumatic defining moments in the past, He will go with me through whatever may come my way in the future as well.

Chapter 14: Honesty Helped When It Was My Turn

Carolyn Evans Shelton's Story as Told to Molly Ford Flodder

After my mom fell in 2017, I visited with the doctor about her general well-being. A young doctor said, "I want you to know that as the result of the x-rays, we can see that your mother has early-onset dementia." I chuckled and said, "Early-onset dementia? That's not bad for being 94 years old!"

Mary Lucille—Lucille, as everyone called her—had done well living on her own for the six-plus years since my dad, Abraham Lincoln Evans died in 2011. She continued to drive for a few years, shop, do the housework, and even learned to pay the bills. Due to her 2017 fall and a urinary tract infection that was discovered in the hospital, she spent a few weeks in a nursing home for rehab. I realized Mom needed more care than I could give from an hour away. She and my older brother, Dick (who lived fairly close to her), did not get along well, and Dick had been dealing with dementia issues for several years but was reluctant to admit it. It was NOT an easy decision, but I decided to move her from Kokomo to Muncie where I could be near her; she agreed. I was thankful to have retired from teaching a few years earlier. This made it possible to help give Mom better care.

In spite of our love for each other, we both knew that her living with us in our home would have been a bad situation. We got her all situated in a nearby assisted living facility with her own belongings, and she liked her cozy apartment. I visited her several times a week, and we talked on the phone every day—at least once. She'd always been a tidy person and took pride in keeping her new "home" orderly. Mom was pleasant, a cooperative resident, and it didn't take long for her to build positive relationships with staff and other residents. She had a great sense of humor, enjoyed having good clean fun, and most always had a smile on her face.

In Mom's 2 ½ years at her "homing center" (as the great-grands called it), her severe osteoporosis caused her to be quite hunched over, and she gradually went from using a cane to a walker to a wheelchair. Due to a fall resulting in a broken scapula, she was a definite fall risk. As weeks and months passed, two more urinary tract infections occurred. The infections caused her to have very scary hallucinations. Once she was on the proper medicine and encouraged routinely to drink and DRINK water, the scary part of the hallucinations subsided.

Mom's memory of the past had always been keen. She and I (and others) would joke about the fact that she could remember every negative detail about everybody. She loved Jesus, and would commonly and pointedly tell others what they needed to do to get right with Him. However, I began noticing that her short-term memory wasn't as detailed.

As I look back now, I believe her "early-onset dementia" escalated after each urinary tract infection. The hallucinations seemed to continue, but the scary part DID NOT. Her eyesight wasn't the best, but she began seeing ants on her couch—first a few, then many, but only at night.

I realized they weren't real when I asked her to describe them. Well, since she said they had just 2 legs I knew... If people came in the room, she'd say, "Don't you see those ants over there?" The response would be, "No, no it's just you and me in here." (After the ANT episodes, Mom decided to sleep in her lift recliner.)

COVID-19 arrived, and over a period of weeks and months. I would remind her that I couldn't come in, and she couldn't go out. It became apparent that she was going to have issues with her immediate environment and "uninvited visitors". They frequently came in the form of children, some being her twin 10-year-old great-grandsons. She generally enjoyed them; they entertained her and kept her mind pleasantly occupied. She would tell them when it was time to leave, and enlisted the staff to do the same. I received a phone call from her, "Carolyn, I don't mind these boys being here, but they wouldn't get a Kleenex when I asked, and they won't talk to me! Where is their mom??"

My approach was to be honest with her. Over the years she's reminded me that I said, "I'll always be honest with you, Mom." When she became insecure about her surroundings, I would say to her, "Mom, you trust me, right? It's very important that you trust me." She would agree. I learned early on how to know which people in her room were real and which weren't. Those who talked were REAL. She and I developed that common ground to help us communicate when I couldn't be with her, and dementia pulled her further from me.

Mom knew her mind was not working as it should. After a questionable situation or visitor, she might say, "Yeah, I know, I know. I'm not thinking correctly. It's not quite right. I remember when I thought that the floor was falling in that night, and I wanted to leave. You were here. I remember." (This was the night I spent with her at her facility trying to calm her before they finally admitted her to the hospital. She was terrified!)

"Yes, but remember? It wasn't real."

"Yeah. But it was real at the time."

At this point in her life—when she was healthy—consoling/informing her with my honesty could bring her back on track.

We had many conversations about what she saw or who was visiting. There was a woman peeking through her "Easter" tree, but she did not talk to Mom. The decorative concrete squirrel we put outside her window didn't talk, but it danced around for her. There were tomatoes growing on the apple tree right outside her window. (I was VERY thankful she had a window in her apartment!) She watched cars in the parking lot come and go. She'd let me know there was a swimming pool behind the fence, and she could see the girls had swim caps on. (There was no pool OR girls.) I reminded her often that neither adults NOR children were allowed to be in her building. During the last few months, there was a small woman, man, and their baby who lived first under the sink in her bathroom and then in her closet. It was sweet to overhear Mom talking to the "cute, sweet baby" as I continued to listen when she forgot to turn her phone off.

As "Covid-19 lockdown" continued, I'm thankful God allowed these friendly "people" to keep her occupied in my absence. I still checked on her, but it was through her window. We both talked on our phones—the windows needed to remain shut; it was often confusing to her. From the outside, I couldn't witness what she was doing, what she was "seeing," how she was interpreting the life around her. These were definitely frustrations for me. I learned that she had slid out of her wheelchair several times, but she didn't appear to be hurt. I was on the phone with her one time when it happened. She pushed her button, and I waited until a helper came. She couldn't get up on her own. And unfortunately, I couldn't be in there.

I knew Mom could not hang her clothes up in the closet; I had done it for her. The staff did her laundry, but she was too humped over to reach up and put things away. Sometimes they would help her. I noticed that her apartment became really messy. There were dirty dishes in/on the sink. She had put dirty clothes on top of the clean clothes in her basket. There was clutter on the floor. I couldn't see in the bathroom. Mom didn't complain. I wondered if, at this point, she didn't notice as much or just knew there was no option. I know the staff was overworked, overwhelmed, and dealt with their own Covid-19 issues. I couldn't be there, but Mom still smiled.

Many times, she understood why I couldn't come in, but other times she would call me and say, "Carolyn, why don't you come, and we'll go out for lunch?" I'd say, "Think about that, Mom," and she'd say, "Oh, that's right. You can't come in." I wrote pertinent information on bright yellow 8 x 11 papers for her to put in different places in her room, such as "Drink water!" A staff member taped them on her TV cabinet, only to have Mom remove "that clutter" the next week.

On March 29—the beginning of "Covid lockdown," my brother died. Mom knew about his dementia and that he was getting worse. I asked if there was any way I could tell her face-to-face. A week later I was allowed to sit outside with her on the porch to tell her. She handled it well although it took some days for her to totally process that her son had died. A couple of weeks later she called me when I was on my way home from Fort Wayne and said, "Carolyn, I want to know what's going on! Dick has been here for a while, so when are you coming?" Needless to say, I was taken aback. I paused, asked God for wisdom, and said, "Mom, what did I tell you about Dick? Is he talking to you?" She thought about it for a minute and remembered that he had died, and he WAS NOT talking to her. We chatted a bit more, and I added: "I'm not really sure why he's there. Maybe he's trying to make up for things or trying to resolve issues." (This was a reference to their long-time strained relationship.) Thinking that he might be there trying to patch up their relationship seemed to pacify her.

My mom was incredibly important to our four sons. They would frequently take turns staying with Grandma and Grandpa. She loved seeing the kids, teasing them, playing with them, and teaching them about Jesus. Over the past years, our oldest, Michael, would say,

"Grandma was a wise, intuitive lady." She grieved deeply when our 2nd son died from a car accident at the age of almost 23. It makes me happy that our boys loved their grandma unconditionally; she was a wonderful grandma to them. When great-grands came along, they were very special to her, too. She would get down on the floor and play with the little ones, even into her 90's. (I'm glad I have many photos of such activities as hardcopy memories.)

Grandsons, Michael, Mark, Mitchell, and oldest great-grandson, Ethan, all saw her in the hospital during her last day. She was not responsive, but they each took some alone time to tell her their good-byes. She passed away 18 hours after arriving at the hospital. I was holding her hand.

A few days after she died, I was told that when a staff member came into Mom's room around 10 p.m. to get her ready for bed she declined and said: "No, I have to wait. Abe's coming to pick me up."

Later she was reunited with her husband of 69 years, AND she was finally able to escape quarantine, ON HER OWN TERMS.

Mom lived a long and full life. She would say, "I don't know what more the Lord has for me to do, maybe to witness to someone." Handwriting became difficult, and she wasn't able to send greeting cards to folks as she had done for years, so I became her "pen." She quite willingly relinquished her bill-paying to me. The decades of being faithful to her/our church had come to a close, as had her Red Cross volunteer job. She still LOVED to talk on the phone, but it was difficult for her to call, and there weren't many old friends left. Over our mother/daughter lifetime, she and I would argue on the phone about all sorts of things, though we shared most of the same values. Even so, it was understood: I had her back, and she had mine. I knew I would miss her when she was gone.

She was a good housekeeper, seamstress, gardener, and cook (...to name a few). I enjoyed our tidy 600 sq.' house and my beautiful Easter dress each year. Her green thumb produced gorgeous roses, AND I inherited her love of candy, especially chocolate! Mom taught me many things, but those that were clearest/strongest at an early age were the values of honesty and trust. We had many conversations about the latter.

Those last 2 ½ years of her life were not easy, but she was a trooper and rarely complained. Having her seven minutes away was a blessing to both of us. It was MY turn to be there for her. She needed me as her advocate and her voice. I wasn't always pleased with the care she was getting (or NOT) and felt that COVID-19 restrictions kept me from helping her. It also made the staff less accountable to residents with dementia AND their caregivers. She was confused on many occasions, but she never forgot who I was. I'm so thankful for that. Maybe I didn't follow the medical protocol regarding dementia, confusion, or hallucinations, but our mutual trust was the rope that often pulled her back to reality. How long this would have lasted, I don't know. She confirmed that I was doing my best for her, and would frequently tell me "What a nice daughter I was." I did not want to live with regrets—she was my mom--I owed it to her. Her last few months weren't easy. She smiled as we celebrated her 97th birthday with pizza, grands, and great-grands, and I'll cherish the photos that prove it, if only through the window.

My advice to others in similar situations? Be there for your parents. Be there BEFORE they need you. Show them you care. If you cannot do it out of love, do it out of obligation, but DO IT, and be the BEST you can be for them. Be their advocate, their voice (and bring them chocolate or something that makes them happy). Make a point to stay in contact with them. Is once a week too much to ask? Set a good example for YOUR children; one day you may need them to be there for you. Mom gave me birth AND gave me advice for 69 years!

It was MY turn to care for her. I miss her so much now that she's gone.

CHAPTER 15: TRAIN RIDE

MARY HARRINGTON'S STORY AS TOLD TO KATIE FREDERICK

I read John Passaro's analogy *Life is Like a Train Ride.*

"Its core proposes passengers get on the train at a certain point in your life, some stay, some get off. Be grateful and cherish those who stay with you. Know at the end, your train will have the right people on it."

Life on the train has its ups and downs.

Seven years ago I had heart surgery. Doctor says, "You have a hole in your heart the size of a fifty-cent piece. Your heart valve is open and will not close." Halloween 2014 — news hits me hard. First reaction was anger — I had lost a bunch of weight and was faithful in exercising. Why now and why me? Was this a trick or treat?

Tests and tests, as the shortness of breath and the pain came and went. My faith is extremely important. Faith helped me stay calm, focused, and strong during surgery day. My husband was anxious, as were my sisters during the extended hours of surgery. I clearly remember going into the surgery suite and asking everyone to pray with me. It was a quieting moment.

I was raised Catholic, attended Catholic schools, and followed the expectations to attend mass six days every week. It was a big part of my life until I left as an adult. My husband and I, at first, didn't feel the need for a church. We taught our two sons respectable principles and ethics. Later I regretted not being part of a religious community.

Both sons, Jason and Kurt, are independent in their belief in God. Jason and his family joined a nondenominational Christian church and invited me to attend. I found Jesus in this wonderful religious environment.

My prayers are thankful that I found Jesus. My children found their path to faith. I pray daily for strength in my life, and pray for others who are having difficulties.

My family is my greatest joy. My belief in God is essential. I have a savior, and I believe I'll go to heaven. Whether time here is long or short, it is now my time to fully define what's important and how I will live my life.

The train ride is a perfect analogy for being alive. I'm now 68. As I look at friends and family, I move forward and I reconnect. Good friends are still good friends. I'm picking up new friends from church. And the train rolls on!

My grandkids say, "We're going to do this and that and everything." They're so focused on their future. I'm just amazed and grateful.

I thought my life was going to be different, but then God altered the plan. On my train ride, I see some of the clutter disembark while old truths remain and new ones come aboard. For every action there is a reaction. From work to home to pleasure to church, I saw actions from and reactions to others.

In my 20s, I spent two years working 25 hours a week, taking care of kids and getting an education. I had to be responsible. I'd go into work at 5 AM and get off at 1 PM, take nursing classes from 1 to 5 at Ball State University, and then go home and take care of the kids and homework until midnight. Next day rolls onward.

This discipline fundamentally changed my life. It made me confident. I'm strong, smart, and proud! When I rediscovered Christ, I felt energized and awake. I was on the right train.

Our church started a ministry in Liberia, a country located along the coast of western Africa.

I was enormously grateful for my life. I was inspired to be taking this eight day excursion with my son Jason. As lists were made for the items to take to the country, at the top were baby formula and water filters. People welcomed us with open arms! Their amenities and life are dramatically different from our country. The people had no access to medicines. Water filters were a critical component. The struggle with dirty water and lack of cleanliness causes much of the diseases in this area. There is just one traffic light for a city of 500,000 people. Nevertheless, the people there have big hearts. To this day, the church continues its ministry three to five times a year to assist with the water filtration tragedy and other issues.

The kids were happy with old soccer balls, boxes, and other small items found. They truly loved to have someone sit down and talk with them. Their smiles were priceless. We sang songs, played kickball, and the kids learned the chicken dance. It was a joy.

It was hard but so rewarding. I stayed calm on the outside. On the fourth night, I broke out in hives from the stress of being there. It was heartbreaking. Daily, I asked God to help me do my work and to get home safely. My prayers were answered.

Now I enrich my life and continue to evolve into the person I envisioned. Marriage, the birth of my children, and grandkids, surviving difficult situations, and getting my education. These are all consistently included on my train journey.

At the end of January 2020, I will have a second heart surgery. This time my heart valve is so tight it doesn't want to open. How will I face it? My answer is: I believe Jesus will be with me, and I know I have the support and love of my family.

Prior to my last surgery, I felt in limbo. Though I feel a bit that way again, I have calmness. Will I wake up with an improved heart or will I wake up in heaven? I do not feel as resilient as I did seven years ago. Mortality is an uncommon thought; thinking about my own mortality is surreal.

My biggest anxiety is how death will happen! There's a funny saying, "I want to go quietly like grandpa, not yelling and screaming like the passengers in his car!" That's what's in my brain — I may never wake up.

My intent is to leave a bit of life that my family will remember. I hope the kids and grandkids will remember the silly and serious Nana and Paps times, remember ups and downs with lessons learned, and realize the beauty around and within each of them. With positive memories, the journey continues. I am grateful for new and old friends who ride the train with me.

Chapter 16: I Was Mad, Real Mad

Rashid Shabazz's Story as Told to River Lin

Mad. Real mad. That's how I feel about racism.

I've been facing racism since the day I was born. Since I was a baby, every day, racism was just a part of life. Bad, unfair things happen to you over and over again and it makes you mad. Real mad.

One time I was at the fair trying to win a Teddy Bear for a little baby. Down to my last quarter and the man in the booth told me, "You get the best 2 out of 3 and you can have any Teddy Bear you want." I said, "OK, I can do that." I got the first one, missed the second one, and then I got the third one.

That man said no. He said I had to get the first 2 out of 3."

I was mad. Real mad.

We argued. Klansmen came around the corner. Crowbars, chains, sledgehammers. All this over a Teddy Bear. Can you believe that? I was thinking how to jump them all: One foot on this guy, another foot on that guy, one hand here, my other hand there.

Then 10 Black men from the community came. One of them said to me, "What's happenin' Lil' Ticket?" Yeah, he called me "Lil' Ticket." Then he said to the Klansmen, "What you gonna do with them toys you got?" I liked it that he called them weapons "toys."

But I was mad. Real mad.

Another time, the Klan set up a table to recruit for new members. Teaching hate. Recruiting so they can do more harm to us.

I was mad. Real mad.

We had a confrontation, and one of those guys had a gun. You can't bring no gun to the fair! And there were all these little kids standing around! Everyone started yelling, "He got a gun! He got a gun!" The police, sheriff, all them came running. That man started shaking, just shaking. I thought he might shoot himself in the leg the way he was shaking.

I was mad. Real mad.

I was one of the greatest basketball players in the country. In the world, really. But racism dogged me so much. By the time I got to high school, I didn't want it no more.

I was just mad. Real mad.

But I was a good player, so they wanted me to be a Bear Cat. I said no, but they got me. See, we had a race riot in the high school and I was right there in the middle of it. Then they gave me an ultimatum: play ball or get kicked out of school.

Oh, no, no. I couldn't face my mother if I got kicked out of school. So I signed up.

But I was mad. Real mad.

In practice I could out-run, out-jump and out-shoot those guys, but in the games, they got all the playtime.

I was mad. Real mad.

Then tournament time came. When we got to the sectionals, we had to play two games in one day, and those white guys, they weren't up to it, so they had to put me in the game.

And I got down!

But you know what? After that, they had to be careful with me because they didn't want a Black hero. No, they'd rather lose with a white hero than to win with a Black hero.

I was mad. Real mad.

And another thing: they only like you when you on the court. During the season, they treat you real good, but after that, they dog you. I went from a thousand people calling out my name and cheering me, to can't even go across the street and have a Coca-Cola or an ice cream cone with them.

I was mad. Real mad.

When I was a senior, the team was on the road, and you know, like teams do, there was some hazing. I didn't do no hazing, but I know who did it. And nothing happened to those white players who did it. But all four of us Black players got kicked off the team for hazing. It was my last year and I was nominated to be Mr. Basketball. That was the real threat; they didn't want me to be Mr. Basketball.

We didn't do no hazing, but we got kicked off the team. I know they just couldn't have a Black Mr. Basketball from Muncie. No title. No scholarships.

I was mad. Real mad.

My anger took me down.

Anger raging inside, my heart was looking for something better.

Religion gave me a white Jesus.

Elijah Mohammed established the Nation of Islam. He preached that the white man was the devil. Seeing how the white man acted, I heard him. I was ready to listen.

My wife had cancer and she passed. The doctors said my baby had it too, and that he needed surgery. I didn't trust them. I read a book by Elijah Mohammed: How to Eat to Live, and it gave me an alternative.

I believed.

I was playing professional basketball by then, but I gave that up so I could care for my son. I got remarried and my wife and I read the Quran to my son every day. Every day. He never had the surgery. He's a grown man now. Healthy. Smart. I'm proud of him.

I believed.

Elijah Mohammed made Black people look at ourselves. He prepared us for Islam. After he died, his son, Imam W. Deen Mohammad, took over as the leader of the Nation of Islam. He preached from the Quran. He preached that there is no superiority among humans, not white over Black, and not Black over white; not Arab over non-Arab, nor non-Arab over Arab. I became a Muslim.

I believed.

Racism is still here. It looks different from how it used to look, but inside, it's still racism. And sometimes, I'm still mad. Real mad.

But today, I'm different because I believe. Oh yes, I believe.

Chapter 17: Michael Brockley Looks Back on His Life Through His Own Words

Aloha Shirt Man Reflects Upon His School Psychologist Career

At first, I wore polyester Mickey Mouse and Garfield neckties. The Disney icon swinging a baseball bat, and the cat cheering the weekend's arrival. One principal complained I was book dumb. A girl who delivered the News Banner told her teacher I was old, fat, and bald. I was 36, listening to "Small Town" on my cassette player. How many bell curves did I scrawl on the backs of scrap paper? How many tales did I tell about Russian nesting dolls and slow cars? Still every time I offered the use of my pencil with all the right answers, the children grinned. I ate apple pies with Flying Jets and Johnny Marzetti with Starfires. Debated Goofy's species with a Raider who watched Pinky and the Brain. For Talk Like a Pirate Day, I knotted a silk Jolly Roger necktie. Pretended a Marvel tie was a school psychologist's cape when Superhero Day was declared. I talked baseball cards with a frightened boy. And exposed the Shawnee Prophet masquerading as Tecumseh. While I visited their classes, crazy-haired teachers in mismatched socks read their students "I'm in Charge of Celebrations." On the 100th day, teachers in old codger garb unveiled the butterfly life cycle to gray-haired children clutching canes. Van Gogh's masterpieces decorated the halls of my schools, beside the hand-printed interviews with giant squids and grasshoppers. When kindergarteners posted graphs of the superheroes they admired, I always found their teachers at the top.

Aloha Shirt Man Thanks the Parents of His Students for Teaching Him Gratitude

You waited for me at the exit where we watched children hustle toward dismissal buses. A few of the third graders already wearing Halloween costumes for the evening's Trunk-or-Treat. You shared a slice of the German chocolate cake your son had baked. Bragged about how he repairs laptops in your neighborhood. Later, worried when your daughter lined up the dinosaurs you bought for her during a trip to the Field Museum in Chicago. She didn't know the worth of a dime, but lectured you on the extinction dates of the pachycephalosaurus. I showed you how to use photographs to teach her; how to brush her teeth. One of your sons gave me a possum doll in a rocking chair for Christmas. A daughter fashioned a birthday collage from National Geographic clippings and orange construction paper. At reading festivals, you fed me Amish meatballs followed by brown-bag apple pie. I listened while you fretted over homework. Questioned discovery math and the latest bell curve myths you heard on the news. I've offered you Kleenex. I've cried alone on my drive home. One spring, I spoke with you about breeding horses during a track-and-field day. On the cinders an Amish boy in farm boots raced ahead of his classmates until slowing along the home stretch to allow three of his peers to win ribbons. Now, I strive to finish fourth in the races I have left to run. I have already won a possum in a rocking chair.

Aloha Shirt Man Thanks the Students Who Made His School Psychology Career a Gift

In the beginning, I showed you how to scramble blocks, and asked what you liked to do for fun. You'd say search for arrowheads in the fields your father plowed. Or play the zookeeper in an Xbox game. When you practiced multiplication facts, I told you how I cheated on times tables tests at St. Gabriel's... until my mother caught me counting on my fingers. I remember the day your social studies teacher forgot Indonesia was an island. The time you taught a substitute the difference between "lightning" and "lightening." You wore green t-shirts with "Pink" scripted on the front or sports jerseys with 18 or 23 silkscreened on the back. I read your recipe for making a peanut butter sandwich, then helped you read *The Grapes of Wrath* in high school. I saluted your graduation from Legos to Minecraft. From Minecraft to the go-carts and guitars you designed during your homecoming year. We amazed ourselves with the shades of red that fall between burgundy and maroon. As the school year closed, I marveled at your superhero shirts folded on the Lost and Found table. At your unclaimed Colts jackets and silver batons. At an unmatched dusty shoe. On my last day, I watched you carry Cat in the Hat kites to waiting cars. Each of you, a knight or a princess, will be the lightning and lightening for all the lives before me.

Chapter 18: Fighting Racism with Love

Mary Dollison's Story as Told to Lauren Bishop-Weidner

Although I was born in Tangipahoa, Louisiana, my memories of the open racism of the segregated South are vague. My mother was very light, but her mother was extremely dark. We used to wonder why our mother was so fair, and her hair was so pretty, and she looked so different from her own family. Well, as we found out much later, her daddy was white. This was Louisiana in the early 1900s, and my grandmother was a domestic worker. She was married, but that didn't matter to her abusive employer. He never did admit my mother or her sister. My mother could have sued her biological father and gotten some of his money, but she didn't want anything to do with that man. She just wanted to get away from the whole situation.

We moved to Muncie when I was 12. My mother worked at Green Hills Country Club, where she met Joel and Inez Reese, both of whom cooked in the dining room there. In addition to that job, Reverend Reese pastored the Kirby Avenue Church of God. Their adopted son, Vernon, was about my age, and even though we were just kids, Reverend Reese trusted us to lead the youth, a role we continued throughout high school. We made some mistakes—bossiness, tattling—but we learned valuable lessons about leadership, discipline, and flexibility. When Cornelius and I married, he joined me in leadership, and we are still working with the kids of Kirby Avenue Church of God all these years later. As a timid young girl with no confidence, working with children helped me to see a little of God's plan, a plan that unfolded gradually.

Around 1956, I started doing domestic work after school and weekends for a wealthy white family who lived near Ball State campus. Despite the racial stereotypes associated with domestic work, that job showed me a future I never could have imagined. I learned to cook a broad array of dishes, to set a formal dinner table, to make small talk with strangers. My vocabulary and my world grew larger from reading their travel magazines, studying the family's fine art pieces, and reading their seemingly endless supply of books. Observing from behind the scenes, I saw what education can do, and I wanted to be a part of that world. With God's help and Cornelius' support, I completed a teaching degree in 1964.

It wasn't easy for a Black teacher to find work in Muncie Community Schools at this time.

Most African-American students were served by either Longfellow or Garfield, and these were the only Muncie schools with African-American teachers. I was given a first-grade class at Longfellow that year, along with three other brand new teachers. I loved working with those women. We shared our lives and our passion for teaching, collaborating in innovative ways to give our students a solid educational foundation. Many of those first graders went on to complete college.

In December 1965, my son Larry was born. When I returned to teaching two years later, Dr. Sam Abram was a rising star in Muncie Community Schools and the only African-American administrator.

Although both Longfellow and Garfield had openings, he strongly encouraged me to request placement in a school serving white students. Three weeks into the school year, I was finally hired at Morrison-Mock. You could say the Dollison family integrated Morrison-Mock – I was their first African-American teacher, and my children were the first Black students to enroll in regular education classes.

When my children faced racism, and they did, I would talk to their teachers. I didn't want special treatment, but I wanted what was right. Each situation was different, and I approached each one as a separate incident rather than as a pattern. At Morrison-Mock, especially in the early years, I sometimes surprised parents: "I didn't know you were Black!" they'd tell me. But children don't see race as adults do. It's our responsibility to demonstrate love and hope and opportunity to ALL children. My great-granddaughter recently asked her mother, "Why are you Black, MeeMee's white, and I'm brown?" She's seeing colors, not race.

In my family, we knew about hard work. We knew you needed to have a garden. We knew you needed to save money. These are good traits to have, but they are not enough. Children need nurturing and encouraging and empowering. Black people understand hard knocks, and sometimes the obstacles we face can make us hard people. If we look at individuals, and treat others as we want to be treated, we can fight racism with love. As my grandmother always told us—I can hear her in my head right now—" You reap what you sow."

Throughout my teaching career, I made a practice of inviting my students to share a meal with my family, a few at a time until everyone in class had a chance to participate each year. As we worked together to prepare the meal and clean up after, we learned about one another, getting to know each other outside of the classroom. The time together offered many teachable moments. We talked about hygiene—handwashing, proper dishwashing. We discussed nutrition: What makes a healthy meal? The children learned new words, such as "condiments." I got to know parents, too, since they had to pick up their children. These individual relationships helped us to trust one another, regardless of race. If we look at the person first and the skin color second, racism doesn't stand a chance.

I'm not a stranger to the ways race can be used against us. But I believe in fighting with love, starting with the children.

CHAPTER 19: DISCOVERING THE PERSON I'VE ALWAYS BEEN

MOLLY FLODDERS'S STORY AS TOLD TO KELSEY TIMMERMAN

The day I announced my retirement, I read the obituaries.

I remember this one lady; it seemed like she had never worked outside the home. It listed what the grandkids called her, and how she loved to make quilts. It was obvious she meant so much to so many and had made a difference in their lives.

I thought about what my obituary might say: "Molly Flodder sure did do a lot of crap!"

When I gave my official retirement notice at the TEAMwork for Quality Living board meeting, I felt good. People said: "Congratulations, you've earned it." Those kinds of things.

But when it finally hit me, I was terrified. I thought, "What am I going to do? Who am I without this work?"

I had sort of gotten into a pattern where I just didn't make time for my friends anymore. They would ask me, "Do you want to go to lunch with us on such and such day?"

"Oh, no," I'd say, "I will be getting ready for a meeting that day."

They had quit asking me, you know, so that was one thing that crossed my mind. What am I going to do with my time?

***

I started working when I was 15, giving piano lessons.

I was married to Mr. Wrong before I married Mr. Right. When I got married one of the things I really wanted to do was get away from home and start my own life. And so, I went to college and graduated in three years. I had four part-time jobs. I kicked it into high gear so I was able to accomplish as much as possible. Gotta move. Gotta do. Gotta get done.

The first part of my career, I was a teacher. I got involved in all kinds of extracurriculars. I was the yearbook and literary magazine advisor. I directed a 90 voice community folk choir of teenagers, too.

And then I ended up at Ball Corp for eleven years. And that was intense in a different way. There was a lot of traveling. I edited the company magazine, and if you're going to write about the plastics plant in Greenville, South Carolina, you got to go down and interview the people. That was a very busy life.

By this time, I was married to Mark, aka Mr. Right. And we had Maggie when I was 35. I was trying to juggle family and work.

I later became the Vice President of marketing and public relations at Ball Hospital. But when I went into healthcare, I didn't know much about healthcare. And so I had a really steep learning curve, and spent lots and lots of hours trying to figure that out. A hospital is a city that never sleeps. If you're meeting with physicians, you might be in an 8 AM meeting and it's your third meeting of the day. I had an average of twenty-three meetings a week. So normal things that moms do to get their kids off to school, I couldn't do.

I think everyone knew I worked really, really hard. And that if I was going to be responsible for a project, or a committee, or a program, I would make sure it got done. I was dependable.

After the hospital, I was the first executive director of TEAMwork for Quality Living, an organization that came alongside people living in poverty. We got started in the mid 90s. I did that for 18-and-a-half years. That was the most exciting, wonderful thing. It didn't even feel like work. I felt like I was making a difference in the community.

I was dreading retirement. I was looking forward to it, as far as, more time and a chance to travel and be with family, but dreading the change in my life and whether or not I'd be able to embrace it, live it, and enjoy it.

I felt like, if you were to line up two lists: one of all my strengths in my working life, and one of my strengths as a wife, mother, friend, etc, the latter would be a much shorter list.

***

There was a time, I hate to admit it, but I might have looked down upon someone with an obituary that didn't include a career. But when I read that lady's, I felt some longing.

It took a good year to settle into retirement.

I actually toyed with the idea of putting a volunteer resume together and sending it out to places. I've cautioned so many friends who are retiring against doing anything like that. Because you don't have a perspective yet to be able to know how much you're going to be able to take on. And so fortunately, I didn't go through with that idea.

I finally came to the conclusion that for me, there's a formula: I can take on two big things where I'm at a central part of whatever is working, whatever's going on, and two or three little things where if I missed a meeting, nobody would think anything. And that works for me.

I don't want to go back to work, but I do believe that this community is important. And it's important to be supportive of younger leaders. And I didn't feel that way for a while. I kind of felt like, you know, they were just a bunch of young kids trying to make sure the old people were stepping on out the door. That's not true at all. If you get to know people and sometimes share something that worked when you were in the workforce, they really appreciate it.

I have my 2021 calendar right here with my goals on it. It's a short list:

Play ukulele. I'm a musician. So I could pick it up really quickly if I just worked on it. My grandkids are gonna be in high school someday. I'm gonna want to sing songs with them now, while they still want to do it.

Read for enjoyment. Don't do that. I was an English major. I love reading. It's my favorite thing in the whole wide world, but I don't do it. Too many household things and lots of community stuff.

Write. I had such a creative imagination when I was a kid. I remember sitting on my bed with my dolls and pretending it was the Mayflower. Giving them names and identities. I could play like that for hours. I don't sit on the bed to play with dolls anymore, but I certainly have the luxury of time to go into my imagination. That's why I wish I were making myself write again.

Compose music. Haven't done much of that for years. Did a little of that with church music several years ago and really hope to do more.

Eat healthier.

Move my body.

I have only started those in the last year due to learning I'm diabetic.

But the last one, I have worked on: *nurture friendships*. I take the time and drop everything to go do something with friends.

I really enjoy hanging out for a full day and not having to put on makeup and not having to go around on a schedule.

I'm psyched to be able to take a nap in the recliner.

When I was eight, we took a trip to Branson. And there was nothing there then, except the small beautiful Ozarks. I enjoyed looking out over the beauty of God's creation.

I've never enjoyed our home as much as I have enjoyed it now. I go outside, look at the river, and appreciate nature. I slow down.

Recently I was sitting outside in a friend's backyard under a huge tree. It's a beautiful spot. We were all just sitting and talking and laughing and having a good time. We meet weekly. I brought one of the dishes for our potluck lunch, and they loved it. We were visiting and laughing. We care about each other.

I want to say something profound here, but my occasionally fuzzy head keeps me from doing very well at that. Retirement was a very strange journey of trying to figure out who I was, and getting to know myself.

After retirement, I think I entered the person I've always been. Retirement has taught me to accept and love where I am.

As for my obituary: I think it would be kinder and gentler now.

My four grandkids call me Moe Moe.

Chapter 20: Facing the Fight: Systemic Racism in Muncie

Cornelius Dollison's Story as Told to Lauren Bishop-Weidner

My parents came to Muncie from Mississippi, after my dad realized that no matter how good a farmer he was, he would never succeed in the corrupt sharecropping system. Bad year, good year, it was all the same with the white landowners keeping the books.

My father got a job in a foundry, and he encouraged his brothers and sisters to come north. I am an only child, but I sure didn't grow up as one—our house was crawling with cousins. One family at a time, relatives would move in with us until they got a check or two ahead and could get a place of their own. Even when they moved out, we all lived close by each other in the Industry neighborhood, not far from where Millennium Place is now. When I was about 12, we moved to Whitely. We continued to host people coming up from the South—my dad always helped the community.

With the move, I transferred from Blaine School to McKinley. At Blaine, I had been enrolled in Algebra, but the principal at McKinley discouraged all Black kids from any college preparatory classes. "Oh, you don't want to do that," he told me, "I'll just put you in General Math."

Looking back you see the racism, all that potential wasted. It's really sad, how the school system kept Black students out of challenging classes, just because of the color of their skin. Algebra or not, I finished school. And my jobs all required me to use the higher math skills he didn't think I could learn.

God granted me favor in my jobs by directing me to people willing to take a chance on a Black man. I was hired on at Westinghouse as an assembler, and then became the first African-American in Production Control. When I put in for that position, the supervisor told me no. I stood there fighting tears, and he decided to give me a chance to prove I could do the work. This was a management position, a real opportunity for me to develop and grow in a job usually reserved for white men. Eventually I transferred to Quality Control, where I did engineering-type testing, calibration, and inspection.

My next job was in the Station Department of Indiana & Michigan Power, overseeing maintenance and new construction. The work was challenging both technically and intellectually. I've always felt very fortunate that they saw my potential as an employee. My last job before retirement was at the GM plant in Anderson. Anderson had the best Process Engineering department of any General Motors plant in the country at that time, and with a lot of innovative new directions. I even got to work on developing the first computer for use in a car.

When I graduated from high school in 1960, African-Americans in Muncie were expected to take menial jobs. We didn't even have Black teachers, let alone Black bankers or managers. But during the 1960s, things started to change. As far as I'm concerned, Rev. A.J. Oliver of Shaffer Chapel A.M.E. gets the credit for opening up employment opportunities for Muncie's Black community. Rev. Oliver operated a lot like Dr. King, gently but firmly guiding civil rights work in Muncie.

We did some picketing of local utility companies and downtown businesses. Rev. Oliver would ask the managers, "Why can't we have some of our girls working as clerks and tellers?" or "You take our money but you won't hire us to work for you?"

Most of the businesses started to hire Blacks—they didn't like that negative publicity—but the manager at Pepsi just wouldn't budge. Rev. Oliver tried all the usual tactics, and during one visit to the manager's office, Rev. Oliver asked if he could use the phone. As he picked up the receiver, he casually asked who the manager reported to, and then called the guy's boss—the president of Pepsi Cola! Pretty soon, Pepsi was hiring us too.

Muncie joined the nationwide sit-in to desegregate Woolworth lunch counters. The store was downtown on Walnut. Three or four of us sat down to order, and the girls behind the counter didn't quite know what to do. They glanced back at the manager, who shook his head, so they said, "We can't serve you here." We just sat there. One whole business day we occupied that counter—and this was going on at all the Woolworth stores across the country! Woolworth's finally relented, and other businesses followed suit. What sense does it make to turn down somebody who wants to spend some money for food?

In those days, the downtown YMCA was for whites, and Black kids hung out at the Madison Street Y. It was a wooden building with an outdoor basketball court on one side and a baseball diamond on the other. Inside we had pool tables and ping pong. I remember when I was little we had a swimming pool. It seemed so big, all that blue water. But when it developed a leak, they had to close it, and we didn't have a pool until Tuhey was desegregated.

Segregation is less obvious today, but it's still there. We had college students just last semester who were warned not to go east of Martin Luther King Boulevard. They felt silly after they got to know the Whitely neighborhood—folks here would help anybody! Law enforcement has a long way to go, too. It's a work in progress, for sure. But one person can make a difference. Rev. Oliver proved that.

Chapter 21: Times to Make a Difference

Jay Zimmerman's Story as Told to Kelsey Timmerman

A few months ago, I thought I was too busy to die. But now I've accepted death. I don't fear dying. I still have plenty to do.

I had asthma as a kid. I remember being in an oxygen tent. I had this doctor, Dr. Jacobs, who bought me one of those old metal toy gas stations and put it together with me in the hospital. He said it wasn't healthy for me to live in New York City, so my parents moved to Florida.

My father found this cottage right on the beach in St. Petersburg. I could literally climb out my window and be on the beach.

During Spring Training, The New York Yankees practiced on my Little League field. It was a different time then. The players were more accessible. Mickey Mantle showed me how to hit. I took a pitch from Whitey Ford. I stood in the batter's box shaking the whole time. Scared the living hell out of me. I didn't swing. I didn't even see the ball.

It was wonderful. It was incredible. It was heaven.

I had a political awakening at 16. Opened my eyes. I was in love with this girl, and she gave me *The Blue Book of the John Birch Society*, a very right-wing group. She took me to a meeting that changed my whole view of things. Members dropped all pretense. The prejudice . . . it was all there . . . out in the open. It was right at the beginning of the civil rights movement. I realized I had to break up with her, which I hated.

In high school, I did a lot of theatre—directing and acting. I won some awards. I would have gone into theatre, but my father and mother said, "No Jewish boy should be going into theatre. You should be a doctor or a lawyer."

My first semester at University of Florida, I got mono. I went home and enrolled at Miami-Dade Junior College. Miami-Dade had a large percentage of African Americans, and I was drawn to them. I met a lot of people reading James Baldwin, a huge influence on my thinking. I remember walking into a bar with two friends, and I was the only white person. It was the first time I had to confront being white. It was a changing point in my life.

The next year I returned to the University of Florida. I was writing for a magazine covering a civil rights rally. The National Guard surrounded the African American neighborhood I lived next to. There were soldiers and FBI everywhere. I went out with friends to take pictures of them. The soldiers and FBI stopped us, surrounded the car, all of these trigger-happy shaking kids who were my age pointing rifles at us. It was scary. And I wasn't brave.

It was Vietnam, and I could have easily been drafted. My draft number was 156. I thought about enlisting in the Navy. But instead, I met with a lawyer in the Atlanta airport. He was a guy who got people out of the draft for $1,500. He told me he could get me out, but I had to agree to do whatever he said. If he told me that I had to pretend to be a homosexual, I'd have to do that. I wasn't ready to have somebody else have that much control over my life. He didn't get me out of the draft. Asthma did.

I didn't know a lot of people who were drafted. I knew people who were getting deferments to go to college. Vietnam was really an unjust war in that way. Most of the people who went didn't have any money or were minorities. You feel two things. Lucky that it's not you. And you feel this unfairness in the system.

I was studying medicine—exactly what my parents wanted me to do—except that I didn't like it. I eventually quit.

I thought maybe I'd be a journalist, so I worked for a weekly newspaper that paid $35 per week. I was assigned to cover a Martin Luther King Jr. speech. I took a friend. It was raining hard. Thank God she had a raincoat because I split my pants and had to use it to cover up. So with split pants, I asked Dr. Martin Luther King a few questions. I felt a little squeamish. It was pretty powerful meeting him.

College was a mixture of being involved in racial protests and anti-war activities. As I look back, my life and action became more focused on social justice, and I became braver and braver over time. Ultimately, I earned a doctorate in psychology at age 25 at the University of Georgia and completed my internship at Ohio State University Medical School. A professor in the human potential movement and expanded consciousness movement guided me as an undergrad. He helped me gain a deeper and more holistic understanding of consciousness, and a more holistic view of the world.

Once you have a consciousness about anything, you can't be unconscious.

I was hired at Ball State and I was doing a lot of diversity work with the Multicultural Center. I felt like I needed some training, and I went to this five-day workshop by Sherry Brown. It was pretty intense exploring yourself and issues.

Sherry would call somebody up who wanted to do work on themselves. So, this lesbian woman said it was very hard for her to be accepting of men because of the way they had treated her. She felt like she trusted me and had me come up. I didn't know whether this was going to be a sort of a collaborative thing or whether it was going to be her screaming at me. We connected really well. She just needed somebody to listen and be accepting of her anger. It felt really significant for her and significant for me. And at the end she said to me, "I want you to make a commitment that when you go back, you'll take an active role."

I said, "Yes." I felt like I had to do it. So when I came back to Ball State, I started the diversity team at the Counseling Center. I started to get involved with the Gay Straight Alliance on campus, which evolved into Spectrum, the LGBTQ group. I worked with a group of students to start Safe Zone trainings that were shared and adopted nationwide at hundreds of universities and high schools.

The woman from the conference . . . amazing that I don't even remember her name. I don't. I looked at the list of people who were there and I couldn't remember.

Being white, privileged, and a man, there are things that I could say that might be harder for other people to say. I remember doing workshops with women colleagues and I would be introduced as Dr. Zimmerman, and they would be introduced as Sharon. I could and did say something about that.

The three things I am most proud of since retiring—Facing Racism, the Arts and Mental Health, and my involvement in Whitely with Food Insecurity, which recently won the grand prize from Neighborhoods USA. I have met and worked with some amazing people. I'd really like to start a fund at the Community Foundation. I want to leave a legacy.

There are times I want to shake people awake to get involved, but I know that wouldn't change their minds. So it's a matter of helping them start to look at themselves. I've tried to start conversations, conversations about diversity.

My whole life has been a part of all these movements.

Phyllis, my wife, and I were involved in United Campuses Against Nuclear War. We did a lot of lobbying. We worked with Earl Conn, a Ball State professor and Quaker. I asked Earl, "How do you do this? It feels like it's a never-ending battle." And he said to me, "God only asks that you try."

I don't believe in God the way Earl did, but that stayed with me. You just have to try. Keep at it. And it's easy to give up, man. It's really easy to withdraw into privilege. There have been times where I have, when the work was just too overwhelming.

Leading up to my retirement party, I had this feeling that nobody was going to come. Maybe everybody thinks that. But it was amazing. Students from years ago came. They put together a book with stories from the hundreds of people I trained—another legacy.

I read all these stories about me and I was like, "Who is this guy?"

While I am dealing with cancer now, and it has been tough, cancer is not my life. I remain active and committed. Social justice is my life, as well as the love of a great family and friends. I especially couldn't accomplish all this without Phyllis.

At one of these hospital stays, it hit me. I thought I was dead. My sadness came over leaving people--Phyllis and my incredible grandkids.

I have regrets, but I mean my life is what it is, and I've come to terms with that. I feel like I've had a pretty significant life. I've made contributions. I feel satisfied. You know, everybody's gonna die.

I told my kids to put me in a canoe, get somebody with a bow and flaming arrow, send me out on the lake. A Viking Funeral.

I have this notion that when you die your energy becomes part of the energy of the universe, and some of your energy forms other life.

I'll be floating out there.

Chapter 22: When the Unrest Came to Middletown

Daniel's Story as Told to Melinda Messineo

Daniel is a pseudonym and he is 73 years old.

Things were so tense at that point in the 1960s. We opened the fire station doors and there was this group of Black men there blocking the exit. They were keeping us from going out on the call and I'll tell you, we were scared. They weren't angry at us in particular. They were just really angry and wanted to let whatever it was on fire just go on and burn.

Another time there was this false alarm where as soon as the firemen were inside the building, a crowd of 75-100 people surrounded the place. The firefighters at the truck radioed for help. It wasn't until officers with a dog came that the crowd was dispersed. There were deliberate fires set, too. There was this one time when we were called out to a small structure fire. It was an outbuilding that was burning, but as soon as we got there, the house on the property just exploded. It burned in a way that houses do when the fire is intentionally set. It was timed to go off when we pulled up. We saw this other house where buckets of gasoline were strung up on hooks with fishing line. Only a small fire would be set but once that line would melt, it was bad news.

And here I was this naïve young white guy, not really understanding what was going on. Who knows who set the fires. It doesn't really matter. Looking back, I see it differently. I know better now why people were upset, President Kennedy was gone, Martin Luther King was gone, and Bobby Kennedy, too. We were part of the authority as some people saw it. The unrest from what was happening in the big cities was making its way here and it was bad.

You see, it wasn't always like this here when we were growing up. We didn't see any animosity in the neighborhood. I grew up in the working-class part of town. It was integrated. In fact, we played baseball together. We never had issues. We were friendly. My dad took us to the dentist on the corner and I never thought about it until later that he was a Black dentist. He was just who we went to. . .never even thought about it.

As we got older, things changed. Going to high school you started to see differences. People were acting differently and treating people differently. Different groups would even use different doors. You could feel the tension; see it in people's eyes.

I remember one day some friends and I went to the carnival down the road. It was one of those mobile ones that would go from town to town. We lost track of time and weren't paying attention to the fact that as white teens, we should have left already. People were nervous that we were there, anxious, upset, deciding what we were doing there still, if they should do something. Things were tense; we knew we shouldn't have been there that late because it made things complicated for everyone. We just got ourselves out of there as quickly as we could and didn't look back.

We all were just expected to stay in our own place. I remember there would be these dances in high school where the white kids would have their record hops which were nice and all, but the dances you really wanted to go to were the live music shows in the armory that the Black community put on. I was lucky because my folks were involved at the armory, so I got to see all the great acts. Otis Redding, Mary Wells, The Drifters, Jackie Wilson, who was the best singer there was—this was before Michael Jackson—and I got to see him, to see all of them. Everyone should have been able to see them but it wasn't that way back then. Things needed to change and they did change, but it was rough.

There wasn't a particular incident that I can point to as the start of it all. We had been isolated, protected from the unrest for a while and I think I know why. What we had then was jobs, and work, and people making a good living, a way to provide for their families. Maybe that's why it took a while for the unrest to come. But I will tell you, I have seen ugliness, an ugliness that only comes from people when they are really afraid. You see, ignorance leads to fear which creates anger which makes hatred. And people, they become sick in a way, unwell, their mental health declines and they become overwhelmed by it all and get so angry. Though I have wondered, and nobody can answer this for me yet, I have wondered, is it the mental illness that causes the hatred or the hatred that causes the illness? Hatred can make you crazy, I have seen it. . .I have seen it destroy people. And it doesn't have to be that way.

You know, you aren't born even knowing what race is. . .it has to be taught to you. . .someone has to tell you people are different and that difference means something. It don't mean something unless someone says it means something, and even then it doesn't really mean anything.

People use it as a reason and as we get older, we need to be careful with our words because the kids are listening, that's how they learn it. We need to work as a community to teach them. It takes all of us together to make a change. And what people don't want to hear is that it is expensive to do it right. It takes time and money and people working together. We are all just too busy. When I was a kid, the police, they had time to mentor to get to know the kids in the neighborhood. Neighbors knew each other. We would help each other out. Now, we don't invest, we don't take the time. I worry now because I see it starting again...the unrest is coming back. It worries me. The Islamophobia is starting here, it's like 1967 all over again. People want to hide and not talk about it, but we have to talk about it, you know? We have to keep talking to each other and build relationships and learn from each other and not be ignorant about who we all are because we can't afford to have that ignorance turn into hatred. It can't happen that way again.

We can't let the unrest come again.

CHAPTER 23: A TIME FOR EVERYTHING

JAMES HILLESON'S STORY AS TOLD TO JACQUELINE HARRIS

Pastor, chaplain, and spiritual educator.

Ecclesiastes 3:1-8

"There is a time for everything, and a season for every activity under heaven:
a time to be born and a time to die,
a time to plant and a time to uproot...
a time to weep and a time to laugh...
a time to be silent and a time to speak..."

This Bible verse is emblematic of how I have lived my life and conducted my ministry. I've often thought that a lot of my awareness of "seasons" came from my early upbringing on a farm. I was born and raised on a farm with two brothers and three sisters. Farm life required a lot of hands on deck, and this produced a strong work ethic. It gave me perspective; there was a strong work ethic and steadiness in our family. When I struggled, I knew I needed to work a little harder. There would be deaths of livestock, a time to die. Additionally, we celebrated holidays and birthdays, so we had times of levity, a time to laugh.

This perspective of birth and death helped my work in hospital chaplaincy as well. Hospitalized people would be going through a difficult healthcare issue, which challenged them, but I was able to talk with them and helped them through their ill-health season. Being hospitalized was only part of their life and they would move into a new season of living. I also brought the idea of seasons of living into my counseling and companioning people as they faced other questions and challenges in life.

How did I get from being an Illinois farm boy to Director of Chaplain Services at Ball Memorial Hospital? I originally thought I'd go into farming, but after two college years, I realized I wasn't the one to take over the family farm. My brother could make good, hard decisions and now runs the farm. I earned a degree in Social Work and then I went into the seminary. I don't know what else I would have done other than go into the ministry. Since seminary, I feel my life has been stretched, my sense of spirituality and faith has widened and been challenged to grow; my sense of being a pastor has changed throughout my life. There would be times to plant and times to uproot, which has helped me during job changes. I've also seen a broader vision of culture and life through my children. I feel God has led me, and as I look back, it has been uplifting and good to feel this was part of God's plan.

One very serious issue I've had to deal with in my ministry is facing a lot of deaths through suicide. It has caused me to think of others' despair and how I can help support other people's journey through life. Suicide is a desperate puzzle that does not give up its answers very easily.

In my hospital work, when I could spend an extended time with people, I'd ask, "What do you regret?" "What do you think about?"

They often talked about people, sending good wishes to or expressing concerns about family members. Pets were also major companions and important to people as well. Another characteristic frequently present was a sense of faith and of a higher power. People would say they wondered how other people got along without a faith in God. Often, people would have a bigger perspective on their illness, which was a way for people to realize they weren't alone. It was common for people to express, "If we pray, let's pray for all those who are worse off than me; pray for people struggling in the world, government, etc."

There was a sense of altruism.

Chaplaincy was hard, but almost every day someone said, "thank you." I've recently retired, but I still have the need to find meaning through helping others. I've signed up to preach as a Sunday morning supply pastor in Marion. I'm also co-chairing an eighteen-month spiritual education class which meets every other month. This has pushed me to read and prepare exercises on a variety of spiritual topics. In my spare time, I volunteer to work on the Cardinal Greenway, help a friend with farm work, and play pickleball. Prior to retirement, I was pushed by a schedule. Now I don't have a schedule. I think differently about "Have to's" now, such as exercising. In retirement, I need to take care of myself so I can do other things I want to do which include gardening, woodworking, etc., so I "have to" maintain my flexibility and strength.

Many people have been influential in my life. My family, including siblings, have been important, and we keep in touch often. Now we compare notes on health and activities. My in-laws have been very accepting. They are good examples of grace, and how to age gracefully. They have been very kind, interested, supportive, and expressed concern to and for me. I've learned many lessons from them over the years. Visits with them leave me refreshed.

My happiest times come with family – camping, times in Oregon, seeing my kids raising their own kids. I treasure those moments when we see our kids being good citizens, being concerned about nature and social issues. It gives me joy to see them being conscientious. Heidi and I feel that we have been fully present as parents.

I think we have flourished wherever we have been.

With retirement, I'm glad I don't have to make as many decisions. However, an issue I'm weighing now is, "If I live 20 years, what decisions should I make now?" I realize that in order to use the remaining time wisely, I need to make good financial and health care plans now.

I have some childhood regrets about miscues and choices, but nothing of serious consequences. Earlier, I had "yens" about things I'd like to do, but now I don't think about them much.

If I were to give my younger self advice, I would say not to be so fearful. I was a little shy and I think it held me back some. The future holds some uncertainty for me as I am concerned about Heidi's health and our kids' welfare. But we are content to stay in this area with the social connections and the resources we have in Muncie.

I know that when helping others in the community and building the family of faith, I am using some of my gifts, and I want to continue to do so.

If I were to pass along a life lesson, especially to my kids, it would be to deepen and broaden their lives. "Deepen," as in finding and knowing their core, their center, what gives meaning. My core is in believing in a God who journeys with me. For my kids, and others, I encourage them to find that which holds them, gives them peace and meaning. To "broaden" is to be open to people of all cultures, faiths, backgrounds, accepting people different from themselves. And to love their families...is vital.

"There is a time for everything, and a season for every activity under heaven."

Chapter 24: Learning From Our Children

Shailla Gupta's Story as told to Clarissa Cheslyn

When I was a child growing up in India, I was taught that when an adult came to your door, you welcomed them in and offered them a seat. It was a sign of respect.

At age seven, a man came to the door and I welcomed him in, just as I had been taught. When my father entered the room, the man immediately rose to his feet to greet my father. As I watched from the corner of the room, I couldn't help but wonder why the man kept standing until my father asked him to be seated.

In that moment, I had this twinge, this uncomfortable feeling deep inside me. I had asked someone from another walk of life, someone that I should have known was "different" in the eyes of my culture, to sit down in my family's home. All at once, I felt the embarrassment that comes from the unknown. I didn't know why it was wrong but I felt a deep rooted acknowledgment that there was a difference between the two of us, yet it was so undefined.

As I reflect on this and the way bias was formed in such an innocent mind; I realize that all biases whether it be social, class, cast, or race are learned behavior. Most importantly, I have realized that what is learned can be unlearned. We, as humans, are not as strong or complete as we would like to think, and by stopping our vulnerabilities from being shown, we let fear become a cancer that grows from within.

One of my fondest childhood memories was learning to knit from our kind and loving neighbor, a Muslim woman. As I was Hindu, I was not allowed to partake in their family meals but that did not stop her from welcoming me into her home. You see, India was and is a land of gentle and gracious people but in the late 1940's partition tore through our country, Hindu- Muslim migration created dividing lines that were fueled by rage and hate. Helpless men became devils and blood saturated both India and Pakistan; but even throughout these trials, the bonds of friendship survived.

When I was just 10 years old, I awoke one morning to see our neighbors gone. Despite the risks it posed to my family, I later came to know that my father had helped them to escape to safety when the risk became too great for them to stay in our neighborhood. In the darkest hours, people still helped each other because we were people, not because we were one religion or another. If in that moment we were able to erase bias, why should it be any different now, living in a country with hundreds of different nationalities and religions all poured into one? Somehow and somewhere racism finds and takes root here, but why?

For me, I believe that racism or any discrimination grows because we are ignorant and we cocoon ourselves out of fear when we should instead be asking and educating. It is difficult for us as adults to break away from these cocoons but luckily we have the ultimate resource available to help us overcome. Children are the ultimate resource in combating this ignorance.

I have come to find that if I am at a grocery store, curiosity will always win over in an interaction with a child. If there is a toddler or a child standing with their mother or sitting on their lap, they will look at bindi–a decorative mark worn in the middle of the forehead by Indian women, and say "Do you have an ouchie?" or they will reach out to touch it. Children want to know. They want to learn, and I want to share. But, the embarrassments from parents who are conditioned to fear cultural embarrassment quickly stifle their child's curiosity. In those moments, they are telling the child not to touch and not to ask and suddenly the child learns that for some reason, I am different.

Years ago I discovered a beautiful quote that spoke to our need to grow outside of our own comfort, it said, "A ship is safe in harbor, but that's not what ships are for." Sure, life is safe in your own little cocoon, never questioning your bias or getting out so you may be exposed to the world's biases. But that is not what this life is for. Life is meant to be lived, to be experienced, and to be shaped by it. As you grow, of course there are challenges. There will be rocks and hidden cliffs in your ship's path, but you will learn to navigate and you will grow stronger because of it.

When I first came to the United States, I was faced with one of the most curious experiences I had ever had with a child. While out in the common area of our university housing, a young girl asked me if I was a witch. I, of course, responded that I was not. She thought for a moment and then asked if I was a Queen. Again, I smiled and said no. Her final line of questioning asked if I was a fairy. As I said no for the final time, the child looked at me and ran away. It was as though she couldn't see the similarities between her and I, so she assumed they did not exist.

These moments are not uncommon and if you have ever walked into a room where you are the minority, you know what it feels like to be me, to be Indian in a community of white faces. You can sense it when everyone wants to look at you and to stare whether it's at a grocery store, the funeral of a close friend, or at a social gala. In that moment you have to make a choice, and I for one have chosen to live and to educate. You have to be willing to know. Be willing to be embarrassed and most importantly, be willing to grow.

SUBMITTED BIOS FOR STORYTELLERS & WRITERS

Michael Brockley has been writing poems since he was a boy with a burr haircut in Connersville, Indiana. Several of his poems have appeared in Facing Project publications.

Clarissa Cheslyn is a Ph.D. student in Health Communication at Indiana University. In her free time, she enjoys writing and performing acoustic shows around Indianapolis.

Julie Davis is a freelance editor who has been working in the Christian trade books publishing market since 2005. Julie and her husband, Clif, have two grown daughters and a teenage son who keeps them busy at the soccer field. In her free time, Julie loves to hike, drink great coffee, watch Agatha Christie mysteries, and read Jane Austen.

Molly Flodder is the retired executive director for TEAMwork for Quality Living, that sponsored the first Facing Project in 2012. In her 44 years in Muncie she has worked in public relations for Ball Corporation and Ball Memorial Hospital. She and her husband, Mark, have two daughters and four grandchildren and are active volunteers in several Delaware County programs and projects as well as at First Baptist Church.

Katie Frederick moved from Iowa to Chicago to Elkhart and finally to Muncie where she entered Ball State University. Katie has worked for various nonprofits, freelanced for anyone who asked. She loves researching and writing! After retirement, she and her husband published two children's books (*Patches and the Delightful Dragon Day* and *The Kite Surprise* – both available on Amazon). They have had great fun reading at schools locally, in Indianapolis and in Iowa.

Ron Groves is an accomplished artist, computer graphic designer, business owner, family man, and community volunteer. For him, at 89 years young, he's been too busy to think about aging itself and continues to work to this day.

Mary Harrington is 70 years old and has lived a great life with many valleys and mountains. She came from a family of eight raised with strong Catholic values but a bit of alcohol and arguments sprinkled within. She has been blessed with two great sons and a husband of over 50 years. She dropped out of college at 20 to be married and have her boys, but she returned at 31 to obtain a nursing degree and start a profession she has been proud to be a part of. She worked at BMH from the age of 19 to 60, but retired due to significant valvular heart issues. She has had two open heart surgeries, and after her second, she had a major stroke. Her stroke, which should have incapacitated her according to the neurologist, was minimal (a bit of memory loss). Mary was very happy to be part of this Facing Project, and hopes those who read it recognize that if you are lucky you will age.

Jacqueline Harris worked in higher education at Anderson University, Ball State University, Purdue University, and Indiana Wesleyan University for 33 years. Upon retirement, she has done volunteer work as an ESL teacher and a Ball State University Rinard Greenhouse docent. She enjoys reading, writing, gardening, sewing, and quilting.

J.R. Jamison is a founder and the president of The Facing Project, and he hosts The Facing Project Radio Show on NPR (produced by Indiana Public Radio). His memoir, *Hillbilly Queer*, was released in 2021.

Brenda Miller is a follower of Jesus and endeavors every day to love God and love others. She's been married to her friend and lover, Eric Miller, for 49 years. She is 70 years old, a mother of two amazing men in their 40s, and a grandmother of two exceptional grandchildren. She loves leading Silver Sneakers at the Muncie downtown YMCA to a group of older adults. She is an active leader in her church. She loves reading and belongs to a couple of book clubs at Muncie Public Library. She also enjoys making birthday cards for her family and friends and taking long bike rides with her husband.

Eric Miller is the husband of one woman, Brenda, for 49 years, which is amazing to him. He is the father of two sons, and the grandfather of two. He is approaching 70 years old. Most of his working career was in manual labor, even though he has a Bachelor's and a Master's degree relating to teaching English. He sees himself as an apprentice to Jesus, and he's thankful He does not fire anyone, because surely, he would have been fired for incompetence long ago. He has much to be thankful for.

Lylanne Musselman is an award-winning poet, playwright, and visual artist. Her work is widely published in literary journals, in addition to many anthologies, internationally. She is author of six chapbooks, and her seventh, *Staring Dementia in the Face* is forthcoming in 2023. Musselman is author of the full-length poetry collection, *It's Not Love, Unfortunately*. Her poems are included in the *Inverse Poetry Archive*, housed at the Indiana State Library.

Donna Penticuff has been a fan of Ron Groves for years, ever since they met when they both were on the Midwest Writers board. She continues to adore him and is pleased to have had this opportunity. She is a former longtime journalist, public relations professional, fundraiser and consultant. In addition, she is a licensed real estate agent. Her most important accomplishment, however, is her family, which includes her husband, three children and five grandchildren. She is facing aging along with everyone else, some days getting the upper hand and sometimes not. Cheers to all as we age together!

John Charles Peterson, M.D.
Family Practice Doctor, Musician.

M. Kay Stickle grew up in Pontiac, MI, and always knew she wanted to be a teacher. College, graduate school, an invitation to join Ball State University: Department of Elementary Education—what fun! There was teaching, consulting, university and community events, and so much more. But nothing like the treasures of life after 60. Volunteering at IU Health Ball Memorial Hospital: NICU, Cancer Center, and ED; Muncie Civic Theatre; High Street U M Church; and Update Learning is so supreme.

Kelsey Timmerman is a founder of The Facing Project and a *New York Times* bestselling author of three books. More importantly, he's dad to Harper and Griffin and husband to Annie.

Jay Zimmerman was a community activist, social justice advocate, artist, writer, retired psychologist, and long-time friend and supporter of The Facing Project. Jay organized Facing Racism in Muncie (2016) and served as the chair of the Muncie-Delaware County Facing Project Steering Committee from 2017 until his death in 2018.

SPONSORS

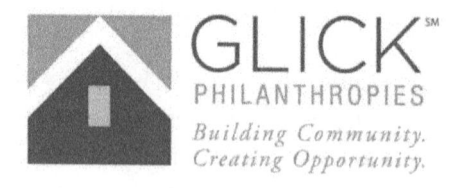

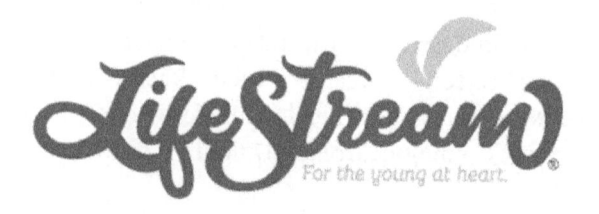

GLICK PHILANTHROPIES
*Building Community.
Creating Opportunity.*

LifeStream
For the young at heart.

the facing project

About The Facing Project

The Facing Project is a 501(c)(3) nonprofit that creates a more understanding and empathetic world through stories that inspire action. The organization provides tools and a platform for everyday individuals to share their stories, connect across differences, and begin conversations using their own narratives as a guide.

The Facing Project has engaged more than 7,500 volunteer storytellers, writers, and actors who have told more than 1,500 stories that have been used in grassroots movements, in schools, and in government to inform and inspire action.

In addition, stories from The Facing Project are published in books through The Facing Project Press and are regularly performed on The Facing Project Radio Show on NPR.

Learn more at facingproject.com.
Follow us on Twitter and Instagram @FacingProject,
and on Facebook at TheFacingProject.

Lightning Source UK Ltd.
Milton Keynes UK
UKHW010730070223
416609UK00002B/526

9 781734 558142